The Washington Manual Internship Survival Guide

The Washington Manual Internship Survival Guide

Written and Edited by

Tammy L. Lin, M.D.
Medical Chief Resident
Former Medicine Resident
Barnes-Jewish Hospital
St. Louis, Missouri

John M. Mohart, M.D.
Internal Medicine Resident
Barnes-Jewish Hospital
St. Louis, Missouri

Kaori A. Sakurai, M.D.
Private Practice
General Internal Medicine
Former Medicine Resident
Barnes-Jewish Hospital
St. Louis, Missouri

Executive Editor

Thomas M. DeFer, M.D.
Assistant Professor of Internal Medicine
Former Medicine Resident
Washington University School of Medicine
St. Louis, Missouri

LIPPINCOTT WILLIAMS & WILKINS
A **Wolters Kluwer** Company
Philadelphia · Baltimore · New York · London
Buenos Aires · Hong Kong · Sydney · Tokyo

Acquisitions Editor: Richard Winters
Developmental Editor: Delois Patterson
Supervising Editor: Mary Ann McLaughlin
Production Editor: Shannon Garza, Silverchair Science + Communications
Manufacturing Manager: Ben Rivera
Cover Designer: Patricia Gast
Compositor: Silverchair Science + Communications
Printer: RR Donnelley/Crawfordsville

© **2001 by LIPPINCOTT WILLIAMS & WILKINS**
530 Walnut Street
Philadelphia, PA 19106 USA
LWW.com

Printed in the USA

Library of Congress Cataloging-in-Publication Data

Lin, Tammy L.
   The Washington manual internship survival guide / written and compiled by Tammy L. Lin, John M. Mohart, Kaori A. Sakurai ; executive editor, Thomas M. Defer.
      p. ; cm.
   Includes bibliographical references and index.
   ISBN 0-7817-3326-X
      1. Internal medicine--Handbooks, manuals, etc. 2. Interns (Medicine)--Handbooks, manuals, etc. I. Title: Manual internship survival guide. II. Mohart, John M. III. Sakurai, Kaori A. IV. DeFer, Thomas M. V. Washington University (Saint Louis, Mo.) VI. Title.
      [DNLM: 1. Internal Medicine--Handbooks. WB 39 L735w 2001]
   RC55 .L56 2001
   616--dc21

                                                        2001016488

Care has been taken to confirm the accuracy of the information presented and to describe generally accepted practices. However, the authors, editors, and publisher are not responsible for errors or omissions or for any consequences from application of the information in this book and make no warranty, expressed or implied, with respect to the currency, completeness, or accuracy of the contents of the publication. Application of this information in a particular situation remains the professional responsibility of the practitioner.

The authors, editors, and publisher have exerted every effort to ensure that drug selection and dosage set forth in this text are in accordance with current recommendations and practice at the time of publication. However, in view of ongoing research, changes in government regulations, and the constant flow of information relating to drug therapy and drug reactions, the reader is urged to check the package insert for each drug for any change in indications and dosage and for added warnings and precautions. This is particularly important when the recommended agent is a new or infrequently employed drug.

Some drugs and medical devices presented in this publication have Food and Drug Administration (FDA) clearance for limited use in restricted research settings. It is the responsibility of health care providers to ascertain the FDA status of each drug or device planned for use in their clinical practice.

10 9 8 7 6 5 4 3 2

Contents

CONTENTS

CONTENTS

Contributing Authors

Dermatology:

Theresa Schroeder, M.D.
Dermatology Resident
Barnes-Jewish Hospital
St. Louis, Missouri

Faculty Advisor:

Michael Heffernan, M.D.
Assistant Professor of Dermatology
Barnes-Jewish Hospital
St. Louis, Missouri

Medical Consultation:

Geoffrey Cislo, M.D.
Former Medical Chief Resident
Barnes-Jewish Hospital
St. Louis, Missouri

Michael Lazarus, M.D.
Former Medical Chief Resident
Barnes-Jewish Hospital
St. Louis, Missouri

Neurology:

Stephen Lee, M.D.
Neurology Resident
Barnes-Jewish Hospital
St. Louis, Missouri

Faculty Advisor:

Richard Sohn, M.D.
Professor of Neurology
Barnes-Jewish Hospital
St. Louis, Missouri

Obstetrics and Gynecology:

Solange Wyatt, M.D.
Obstetrics and Gynecology Resident
Barnes-Jewish Hospital
St. Louis, Missouri

Faculty Advisor:

David Cohn, M.D.
Assistant Professor of Obstetrics
    and Gynecology
Barnes-Jewish Hospital
St. Louis, Missouri

Ophthalmology:

Samir Sayegh, M.D.
Ophthalmology Resident
Barnes-Jewish Hospital
St. Louis, Missouri

Faculty Advisor:

Jonathon Silbert, M.D.
Assistant Professor of
    Ophthalmology and
    Visual Sciences
Barnes-Jewish Hospital
St. Louis, Missouri

Otolaryngology:

Christopher Yian, M.D.
Otolaryngology Resident
Barnes-Jewish Hospital
St. Louis, Missouri

Faculty Advisor:

Mark Wallace, M.D.
Assistant Professor of Otolaryn-
    gology
Barnes-Jewish Hospital
St. Louis, Missouri

Psychiatry:

David Montani, M.D.
Fellow, Forensic Psychiatry
Former Psychiatry Chief
    Resident
Chicago, Illinois

CONTRIBUTING AUTHORS

Radiology:

Ronald Gerstle, M.D.
Radiology Resident
Mallinkrodt Institute of Radiology
Barnes-Jewish Hospital
St. Louis, Missouri

General Surgery:

Ernest Franklin, M.D., MBA
General Surgery Resident
Barnes-Jewish Hospital
St. Louis, Missouri

Faculty Advisor:

Gerald Doherty, M.D.
Professor of Surgery
Barnes-Jewish Hospital
St. Louis, Missouri

Orthopaedic Surgery:

Raja Dhalla, M.D.
Orthopaedic Surgery Resident
Barnes-Jewish Hospital
St. Louis, Missouri

Faculty Advisor:

David Miller, M.D.
Associate Professor of Ortho-
    paedic Surgery
Barnes-Jewish Hospital
St. Louis, Missouri

Preface

This is a pocket-sized companion *survival guide* written and edited by former and current Washington University residents (all former interns). It is meant to be complementary to *The Washington Manual of Medical Therapeutics* and *The Washington Manual of Ambulatory Therapeutics* and to contain concise and practical information for those learning the basics of practicing clinical medicine. It is written assuming basic knowledge of pathophysiology and data interpretation. The target audience is primarily those beginning their internship, but this guide will be useful for medical students, residents, and anyone else on the front lines of patient care.

A deliberate attempt was made to keep the format succinct so the information you need and other hard-to-find material are always available in a rapidly accessible format. It also includes essential *what not to miss* and *when to call for help* information for those who really do need to know what to do when faced with an unfamiliar situation. In short, it's what we wished we'd had, in one reference, when we were interns. It is written assuming that a standard textbook of internal medicine, the *Washington Manuals*, *Sanford Guide*, *Physicians' Desk Reference*, and Internet access (as well as your resident) are available nearby for reference.

T. L. L.
J. M. M.
K. A. S.

Acknowledgments

We wish to thank the following reviewers (many from the 2000–01 intern class at Washington University) for their thoughtful comments that have made our guide immeasurably better: Michael Barry, M.D.; Douglas Bree, M.D.; David Brody, M.D.; Richard Garmany, M.D.; Evan Gross, M.D.; J. Langston Hoffman, M.D.; Grace Lin, M.D.; Robert Makar, M.D., Ph.D.; Melissa Norton, M.D.; Chris Pavlovic, M.D.; Michael Riley, M.D.; Jason Rothschild, M.D.; Scott Rypkema, M.D.; Gregory Sayuk, M.D.; Chirag Shah, M.D.; and Megan Wren, M.D.

For their support and assistance, we wish to thank Gregory Golladay, M.D.; Daniel Goodenberger, M.D.; Wendy Houston; Jacqueline Howard, M.D.; Grace Lin, M.D.; Howard Lu (especially for technical assistance); Leo MacDonald, Jr.; Janet Mueller, R.N.; Kenneth Polonsky, M.D.; Lynn Telfair; Alison Whelan, M.D.; Eric White, M.D.; and David Windus, M.D.

From Silverchair Science + Communications, we are grateful to Elizabeth Willingham and particularly Shannon Garza for their patience and able assistance.

From Lippincott Williams & Wilkins, we wish to thank Sarah Kane, Kathy Neely, Delois Patterson, Mary Ann McLaughlin, and Richard Winters for his steadfast support and expert guidance.

We would like to extend our gratitude to Dr. Thomas DeFer for his encouragement, editorial expertise, and dedication to teaching us and others before us.

For their support and understanding, we wish to thank our families, especially Howard Lu, Susan Mohart, and Brian Kearns.

Abbreviations List

AAA = abdominal aortic aneurysm
AMA = against medical advice
AP = anteroposterior
APC = atrial premature contraction
ARF = acute renal failure
ATN = acute tubular necrosis
AVNRT = AV nodal reentrant tachycardia
AVRT = atrioventricular reciprocating tachycardia
BBB = bundle branch block
BP = bullous pemphigoid
CAD = coronary artery disease
CHF = congestive heart failure
COPD = chronic obstructive pulmonary disease
CPAP = continuous positive airway pressure
CXR = chest x-ray
D/C = discharge
DKA = diabetic ketoacidosis
ECF = extracellular fluid
FFP = fresh frozen plasma
GERD = gastroesophageal reflux disease
GN = glomerulonephritis
H & P = history and physical examination
β-hCG = human chorionic gonadotropin-β
Hct = hematocrit
HEENT = head, eyes, ears, nose, and throat
HTN = hypertension
I/O = input/output
JPCs = junctional premature contractions
JVP = jugular venous pulse
LBBB = left bundle branch block
LMWH = low-molecular-weight heparin
LP = lumbar puncture
LVH = left ventricular hypertrophy
NS = normal saline
NSAID = nonsteroidal antiinflammatory drug
NSR = normal sinus rhythm
PA = posteroanterior
PE = physical examination
PICC = peripherally inserted central catheter
PID = pelvic inflammatory disease
PUD = peptic ulcer disease

ABBREVIATIONS LIST

PV = pemphigus vulgaris
PVC = premature ventricular contraction
RR = respiratory rate
RTA = renal tubular acidosis
SBO = small bowel obstruction
SBP = systolic BP
SJS = Stevens-Johnson syndrome
SOB = shortness of breath
T = temperature
TDP = torsades de pointes
TIA = transient ischemic attack
TSH = thyroid-stimulating hormone
TSS = toxic shock syndrome
UTI = urinary tract infection
VPC = ventricular premature contraction

1 Keys to Survival

. . . Or how to NOT get voted off of the island . . .

1. Don't panic.

2. Take care of your patients. You are finally using your education and training.

3. Be kind to the nurses. They can make your life much better . . . or much worse.

4. Sleep when you can.

5. Remember to eat.

6. Ask for help.

7. Wear comfortable shoes.

8. Call your significant other when on-call.

9. Ask questions. Believe it or not, you are not expected to know everything.

10. Call in consultations on your patients early in the day. This is always appreciated.

11. Start thinking about discharge/disposition planning from day 1.

12. When generating a differential diagnosis, look for an etiology in VITAMIN E:
    *V*ascular, *I*nfection/*I*nflammatory, *T*rauma, *A*cquired/*A*utoimmune, *M*etabolic/*M*edications, *I*nherited/*I*atrogenic/*I*diopathic, *N*eoplastic, *E*nvironmental

13. Work hard, stay enthusiastic, and maintain interest!

2 ACLS Algorithms

. . . First, take a deep breath. Second, take your own pulse. Now you can begin worrying about the patient . . .

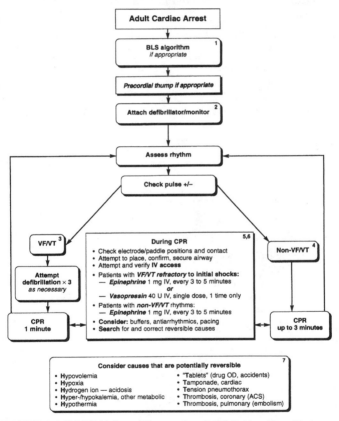

FIGURE 2-1. ILCOR Universal/International ACLS Algorithm. (From Guidelines 2000 for cardiopulmonary resuscitation and emergency cardiovascular care. Part 6: advanced cardiovascular life support: 7C: a guide to the International ACLS algorithms. The American Heart Association in collaboration with the International Liaison Committee on Resuscitation. *Circulation* 2000;102[Suppl 8]:I-143, with permission.)

FIGURE 2-2. Comprehensive ECC Algorithm. (From Guidelines 2000 for cardiopulmonary resuscitation and emergency cardiovascular care. Part 6: advanced cardiovascular life support: 7C: a guide to the International ACLS algorithms. The American Heart Association in collaboration with the International Liaison Committee on Resuscitation. *Circulation* 2000;102[Suppl 8]:I-144, with permission.)

FIGURE 2-3. Ventricular Fibrillation/Pulseless VT Algorithm. (From Guidelines 2000 for cardiopulmonary resuscitation and emergency cardiovascular care. Part 6: advanced cardiovascular life support: 7C: a guide to the International ACLS algorithms. The American Heart Association in collaboration with the International Liaison Committee on Resuscitation. *Circulation* 2000;102[Suppl 8]:I-147, with permission.)

Pulseless Electrical Activity Algorithm

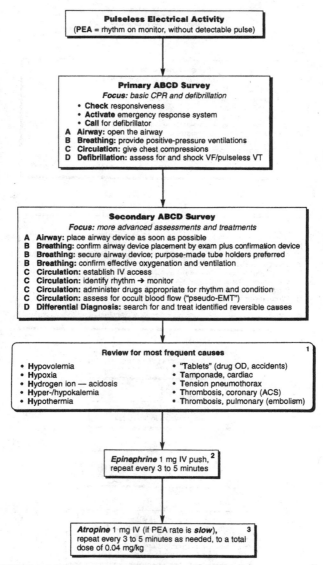

FIGURE 2-4. Pulseless Electrical Activity Algorithm. (From Guidelines 2000 for cardiopulmonary resuscitation and emergency cardiovascular care. Part 6: advanced cardiovascular life support: 7C: a guide to the International ACLS algorithms. The American Heart Association in collaboration with the International Liaison Committee on Resuscitation. *Circulation* 2000;102[Suppl 8]:I-151, with permission.)

FIGURE 2-5. Asystole: The Silent Heart Algorithm. (From Guidelines 2000 for cardiopulmonary resuscitation and emergency cardiovascular care. Part 6: advanced cardiovascular life support: 7C: a guide to the International ACLS algorithms. The American Heart Association in collaboration with the International Liaison Committee on Resuscitation. *Circulation* 2000;102[Suppl 8]:I-153, with permission.)

FIGURE 2-6. Bradycardia Algorithm. (From Guidelines 2000 for cardio-pulmonary resuscitation and emergency cardiovascular care. Part 6: advanced cardiovascular life support: 7C: a guide to the International ACLS algorithms. The American Heart Association in collaboration with the International Liaison Committee on Resuscitation. *Circulation* 2000;102[Suppl 8]:I-156, with permission.)

FIGURE 2-7. The Tachycardia Overview Algorithm. (From Guidelines 2000 for cardiopulmonary resuscitation and emergency cardiovascular care. Part 6: advanced cardiovascular life support: 7D: the tachycardia algorithms. The American Heart Association in collaboration with the International Liaison Committee on Resuscitation. *Circulation* 2000; 102[Suppl 8]:I-159, with permission.)

Narrow-Complex Supraventricular Tachycardia Algorithm

FIGURE 2-8. Narrow-Complex Supraventricular Tachycardia Algorithm. (From Guidelines 2000 for cardiopulmonary resuscitation and emergency cardiovascular care. Part 6: advanced cardiovascular life support: 7D: the tachycardia algorithms. The American Heart Association in collaboration with the International Liaison Committee on Resuscitation. *Circulation* 2000;102[Suppl 8]:I-162, with permission.)

FIGURE 2-9. Stable Ventricular Tachycardia (Monomorphic or Polymorphic) Algorithm. (From Guidelines 2000 for cardiopulmonary resuscitation and emergency cardiovascular care. Part 6: advanced cardiovascular life support: 7D: the tachycardia algorithms. The American Heart Association in collaboration with the International Liaison Committee on Resuscitation. *Circulation* 2000;102[Suppl 8]:I-163, with permission.)

3

Accumulating Your War Chest

. . . A good offense is the best defense . . .

BOOKS AND TOOLS TO CARRY WITH YOU

Most house officers carry a compact general manual of internal medicine in their pocket. Any of the following are useful and practical:

- Ahya S, Flood K, Paranjothi P, eds. *The Washington manual of medical therapeutics*, 30th ed. Philadelphia: Lippincott Williams & Wilkins, 2001.
- Ferri FF, ed. *Practical guide to the care of the medical patient*, 4th ed. St. Louis: Mosby, 1998.
- Gomella LG, ed. *Clinician's pocket reference*, 8th ed. Stamford, CT: Appleton & Lange, 1997.
- Marshall SA, Ruedy J, eds. *On call principles and protocols*, 3rd ed. Philadelphia: WB Saunders, 2000.
- Dubin D, ed. *Rapid interpretation of EKG's*, 5th ed. Tampa, FL: Cover Publishing Company, 2000. (Okay, so it's not likely that you're going to carry this around with you, but it's a great resource to keep in your locker or backpack.)

Other small pocket guides you don't want to be without:

- *Tarascon pocket pharmacopoeia 2001*. Loma Linda, CA: Tarascon Publishing, 2001.
- Rollings RC, Erica T, eds. *Facts and formulas*. Saline, MI: McNaughton & Gunn, 1984.
- Gilbert DN, Moellering RC, Sande MA, eds. *The Sanford guide to antimicrobial therapy*. Hyde Park, VT: Antimicrobial Therapy Inc, 2001.

Other things to carry with you:

- A good stethoscope
- Reflex hammer
- Guaiac developer
- Vacutainer hub
- Ophthalmoscope/otoscope (Yes, you still need this; make sure it's charged for your call and leave it in your locker.)
- ABG kit

HANDHELD COMPUTER RESOURCES
. . . All in the palm of your hand . . .

Drug References

- ePocrates
  Free drug reference updates via AvantGo every time you HotSync
  www.epocrates.com

Calculations

- MedMath
  A useful medical calculator (A-a gradient, BMI, cardiac output, etc.)
  http://mail.med.upenn.edu/~pcheng/medmath/
- MedCalc
  http://netxperience.org/medcalc/index2.html
- ABGPro
  Neat ABG analyzer
  www.bigfoot.com/~wcarlson

Data Tracking

- Patient Keeper
  Electronic patient tracking system for your PalmPilot
  www.patientkeeper.com
- Pocket MD
  www.pocketmed.org

Other Useful Sites

- K2 Products
  The home of Apothecarium, 5 Minute Clinical Consult, and Lexi-drugs (all are for purchase)
  www.skyscape.com
- Avantgo
  Download great Web sites to your PalmPilot, you've got to have this!
  www.avantgo.com
- PDA MD
  Comprehensive site with news reviews, columns, forums, tutorials, and products
  www.pdamd.com
- Your institution's house staff homepage may allow you to download useful things like pager numbers, e-mail addresses, and a weekly conference schedule.

INTERNET RESOURCES

. . . Unfortunately, sleep is not downloadable at this time. . . .

General Sites (Contain Information on a Variety of Problems)

health.yahoo.com
www.medscape.com (Medscape)
www.guideline.gov (National Guidelines Clearinghouse)
www.ama-assn.org (American Medical Association)
www.healthfinder.gov (Department of Health and Human Services)
www.mayohealth.org (Mayo Clinic)
www.mdconsult.com (MD Consult; fee required)
www.acponline.org (American College of Physicians)

Cardiovascular Disease

www.americanheart.org (American Heart Association)
www.nhlbi.nih.gov (National Heart, Lung, and Blood Institute)
www.heartinfo.org (Heart Information Network)
www.acc.org (American College of Cardiology)

Cerebrovascular Disease and Stroke

www.mayo.edu/cerebro/education/stroke.html (Mayo Clinic)
www.ninds.nih.gov (National Institute of Neurological Diseases)
www.stroke.org (National Stroke Foundation)
www.neuro.wustl.edu/stroke (Washington University)

Pulmonary Diseases and Allergy

www.emphysemafoundation.org (National Emphysema Foundation)
www.aafa.org (Asthma and Allergy Foundation of America)
www.sleepapnea.org (American Sleep Apnea Association)
www.chestnet.org (American College of Chest Physicians)

Endocrine and Diabetes

www.niddk.nih.gov (National Institute of Diabetes and Digestive and Kidney Diseases)
www.diabetes.org (American Diabetes Association)
www.endo-society.org (The Endocrine Society)
www.thyroid.org (American Thyroid Association)

Rheumatology

www.arthritis.org (The Arthritis Foundation)
www.lupus.org (Lupus Foundation of America)
www.nih.gov/niams (National Institute of Arthritis and Musculoskeletal and Skin Diseases)
www.rheumatology.org (American College of Rheumatology)

Nephrology

www.niddk.nih.gov (National Institute of Diabetes and Digestive and Kidney Diseases)
www.renalnet.org (RenalNet—Kidney Information Clearinghouse)
www.kidney.org (National Kidney Foundation)

Oncology

www.cancer.org (American Cancer Society)
www.nci.nih.gov (National Cancer Institute)
www.oncolink.upenn.edu (University of Pennsylvania)
cancertrials.nci.nih.gov (National Cancer Institute—Clinical Trials)

Gastroenterology

www.gastro.org (American Gastroenterological Association)
www.acg.gi.org (American College of Gastroenterology)
www.ccfa.org (Crohn's and Colitis Foundation of America)

Infectious Disease/HIV

hivinsite.ucsf.edu (University of California at San Francisco—HIV site)
www.cdc.gov (Centers for Disease Control and Prevention)
www.niaid.nih.gov (National Institute of Allergy and Infectious Diseases)
www.who.int (World Health Organization)

Geriatrics, Aging, Osteoporosis

www.alzheimers.org/adear (Alzheimer's Disease and Referral)
www.aoa.dhhs.gov/elderpage.html (Administration on Aging)
www.osteo.org (National Institutes of Health—Osteoporosis and Related Bone Diseases—National Resource Center)

Women's Health

www.4woman.gov (National Women's Health Information Center)
www.womens-health.com (Women's Health Interactive)
www.womens-health.org (Society for Women's Health Research)
www.wellweb.com/WOMEN/WOMEN.HTM

Online Journals

www.acponline.org/journals/annals/annaltoc.htm (Annals of Internal Medicine)
www.bmj.org (British Medical Journal)
www.jama.ama-assn.org (JAMA—Journal of the American Medical Association)
www.thelancet.com (The Lancet)
www.nejm.org (New England Journal of Medicine)

Online Pharmacies

www.cvs.com (CVS)
www.drugstore.com (Drugstore)
www.planetrx.com (Planet Rx)

INTERNET RESOURCES FOR
EVIDENCE-BASED MEDICINE

The Cochrane Database of Systematic Reviews:
http://cochranelibrary.net

Reviews, analyzes, and synthesizes the best clinical trials by topics.
Multi-directional links MEDLINE, EBM, and EUCLID full-text.

Pubmed: http://www.nlm.nih.gov

Maintained by the National Library of Medicine
Allows a user-friendly approach to medical literature with built-in
search filters.

ACP Journal Club

http://www.acponline.org/journals/acpjc/jcmenue.htm

4

Useful Formulas

... CORRECTED SLEEP EQUATION ...

$$Sleep\ (hrs)\ =\ \frac{[Discharges + Transfers]}{[Admissions + Cross\text{-}cover]^2} \times Interns$$

A-a O$_2$ GRADIENT

- $PAO_2 = (FIO_2 \times 713) - \left(\dfrac{PaCO_2}{0.8}\right)$
- A-a gradient = $PAO_2 - PaO_2$
- Correction of gradient for age 2.5 + 0.25 (age)
  Normal = 3–16 (<8 if younger than 30 years old)

Causes of Increased A-a Gradient

- $\dot{V}/\dot{Q}$ mismatch
- Intrapulmonary right-to-left shunt
- Intracardiac right-to-left shunt
- Impaired diffusion (room air only)

ANION GAP (SERUM)

- AG = [Na] – ([Cl] + [HCO$_3$])
  Normal = 8–12 mEq/L
  See Acid-Base section in Chapter 16 for differential diagnosis.

ANION GAP (URINE)

- UAG = (U[Na] + U[K]) – U[Cl]
  Normal = slightly positive
- UAG is **negative** in diarrhea-induced non-gap metabolic acidosis
  (**enhanced** urinary NH$_4$ excretion).
- UAG is **positive** in distal RTA–induced non-gap metabolic acidosis
  (**impaired** urinary NH$_4$ excretion).

BODY MASS INDEX

$$BMI\ =\ \frac{weight\ (kg)}{height\ (m)^2}\quad or \quad \frac{weight\ (lb)}{height\ (in)^2} \times 704.5$$

<19, underweight
19–25, normal weight
25–30, overweight
>30, obese

CREATININE CLEARANCE

- $CrCl = U[Cr] \times \dfrac{\text{urine volume}}{P[Cr]} \times \text{time}$

  Creatinine in mg/dL, volume in mL, and time in minutes
  Normal CrCl >100 mL/min

CREATININE CLEARANCE (ESTIMATED)

$CrCl = (140 - \text{age}) \times \dfrac{Wt}{72} \times P[Cr]$

For women, multiply the result by 0.85
Weight in kilograms, creatinine in milligrams per deciliter

CORRECTED SERUM CALCIUM

Corrected serum Ca = measured [Ca] + [0.8 (4.0 – measured albumin)]

CORRECTED SERUM SODIUM

Corrected serum Na = measured [Na] + [.016 × (measured [glucose] – 100)]

FRACTIONAL EXCRETION OF SODIUM

$FENa = \dfrac{U[Na]}{P[Na]} \times \dfrac{P[Cr]}{U[Cr]} \times 100$

FENa <1% in prerenal states; not valid when diuretics have been given

FRACTIONAL EXCRETION OF UREA

$FEurea = \dfrac{U[urea]}{BUN} \times \dfrac{P[Cr]}{U[Cr]} \times 100$

FEurea <35% in prerenal states; not affected by diuretics

MEAN ARTERIAL PRESSURE

$MAP = \dfrac{SBP + (2 \times DBP)}{3}$

OSMOLALITY (SERUM, ESTIMATED)

Calculated serum osmolality = $(2 \times [Na]) + \dfrac{\text{glucose}}{18} + \dfrac{BUN}{2.8}$

OSMOLAL GAP

Osmolal gap = measured S_{osm} – calculated S_{osm}

Causes of Increased Osmolal Gap

Decreased serum water
    Hyperproteinemia
    Hypertriglyceridemia
Presence of unmeasured osmoles
    Sorbitol, glycerol, mannitol, ethanol, isopropyl alcohol, acetone,
        ethyl ether, methanol, and ethylene glycol

RETICULOCYTE INDEX

$$\text{Reticulocyte index} = \frac{\text{reticulocyte count} \times \text{Hct (measured)}}{45\% \text{ (normal Hct)}}$$

- The reticulocyte count is not accurate in anemia, so use the reticulocyte index.
- Good marrow response = 2.0–6.0.
- Normal <2.

MEDICAL EPIDEMIOLOGY

Test Result	Disease	No Disease
Positive	True positive	False positive
	(A)	(B)
Negative	False negative	True negative
	(C)	(D)

- **Sensitivity:** The percentage of patients with the target disorder who have a positive result (A/[A + C]). The greater the sensitivity, the more likely the test will detect patients with the disease. High sensitivity tests are useful clinically to rule out a disease (SnOUT) (i.e., a negative test result would virtually exclude the possibility of the disease).
- **Specificity:** The percentage of patients without the target disorder who have a negative test result (D/[B + D]). Very specific tests are used to confirm or rule in the presence of disease (SpIN).
- **Positive predictive value (PPV):** The percentage of persons with positive test results who actually have the disease (A/[A + B]).
- **Negative predictive value (NPV):** The percentage of persons with negative test results in which the disease is absent (C/[C + D]).
- **Number needed to treat (NNT):** The number of patients who need to be treated to achieve one additional favorable outcome; calculated as 1/absolute risk reduction (ARR), rounded up to the nearest whole number.
- **Number needed to harm (NNH):** The number of patients who, if they received the experimental treatment, would lead to one additional person being harmed compared with patients who receive the control treatment; calculated as 1/absolute risk increase (ARI).

Triage

BEFORE ACCEPTING ADMISSIONS

. . . Do ask, do tell . . .

1. Obtain vital stats: name, date of birth, medical record number.
2. Why does the patient need to be admitted to your service?
3. Is the patient competent and does he or she want to be admitted?
4. What are the patient's chief complaints, comorbidities, relevant past medical history, and brief history?
5. When was the last previous admission? Obtain old medical records (inpatient and outpatient).
6. Obtain vital signs, pertinent examination including mental status, key lab data, CXR, ECG, code status. Review as many lab results and films in the ER as you can.
7. Confirm IV access.
8. Inquire about major interventions performed, consultations pending.
9. What follow-up is necessary (i.e., lab tests that are pending, consults that need to be called, blood transfusions, antibiotics)?
10. Find out who is the accepting primary MD and if this person has been notified.
11. Do family members need to be called?

OTHER IMPORTANT QUESTIONS TO CONSIDER

. . . Location, location, location . . .

- Is this an appropriate admission for your service (i.e., is there something you can do for the patient that no one else can do? Does a different service make more sense?)?
- Can this patient be managed as an outpatient? If yes, social services may need to be involved. In addition, arranging follow-up is crucial.
- Is the patient stable enough for the floors? Are any more treatments needed before transfer to the floor (i.e., nebulizer treatments, etc.)?
- Can your staff adequately handle this patient?
- What specific interventions does this patient need that other institutions cannot provide (in the case of a hospital-to-hospital transfer)?
- Obtain collateral information from family, nursing homes, or other caregivers. Always collect and hold onto important phone contacts.

6

Cross-Coverage

. . . Who? What? Wait, let me get my sign-out . . .

GENERAL POINTS

1. For the first few months of residency, when you are called about a patient, it is a good idea to go see the patient and assess the situation. This should be until you feel comfortable deciding what situations can be adequately handled over the telephone with the nurses and the support staff.
2. Always go see the patient if you have any doubt or concern. The patient is always your number one priority.
3. If you do go see a patient, always write a note (this can be brief, depending on the situation). Things to document include
   A. Reason you were called to see patient (i.e., CTSP for chest pain).
   B. Assessment of situation on arrival including general appearance, vitals, pertinent physical examination.
   C. Interventions.
   D. Outcome.

REASONS YOU MUST GO SEE A PATIENT

. . . Drop everything and go now. Godspeed . . .

1. Any major changes in clinical status
   • Altered mental status or other changes in neurologic state
   • Dyspnea
   • Chest pain
   • Severe abdominal pain
   • Seizures
   • Uncontrolled bleeding (hemoptysis, hematemesis, lower GI bleed)
   • Uncontrolled vomiting
   • Severe headache
   • New onset of pain
2. Any major changes in vital signs
   • Oxygen desaturation
   • Hypotension
   • Arrhythmias (tachyarrhythmias and bradyarrhythmias)
   • Fever associated with changes in mental status, changes in vital signs

THINGS TO CONSIDER ASKING FOR BEFORE ARRIVAL AT BEDSIDE

. . . Delegate before it's too late . . .

1. Full set of vitals.
2. Hospital chart at bedside.

3. IV access.
4. Oxygen (nasal cannula, face mask), respiratory therapist.
5. Cardiac monitor, ECG.
6. Crash/code cart.
7. Chest x-ray.
8. ABG kits.
9. Blood cultures, if febrile.
10. Basic lab results.
11. Restraints.
12. In situations in which the patient is becoming unstable and you are having difficulty, have the resident paged immediately!

THINGS THAT CAN WAIT

. . . Passing back the pain . . .

1. Talking to family members, unless urgent; this can usually be handled by the primary team.
2. Major adjustments in medication regimen in a stable patient (i.e., diabetic medicines, antihypertensive medicines, antibiotics).
3. Consultations in nonemergent, stable situations (i.e., GI consult in patient with Hemoccult-positive brown stool, stable hematocrit, stable vital signs).
4. Renewal of restraints/telemetry orders.
5. Addressing code status in a stable patient.

APPROPRIATE TRANSFER OF PATIENTS TO THE INTENSIVE CARE UNIT

. . . Passing on the pain . . .

1. Determine which unit is most appropriate for management of the patient.
2. Speak to the resident who will be accepting the patient to inform him or her of the situation.
3. Have the nursing staff give report to the staff in the unit.
4. Every patient needs a brief transfer note, including:
   A. When and why you were called to see the patient.
   B. One-line description of patient and his or her comorbidities.
   C. Your assessment of the situation.
   D. Your management of the situation, including diagnostic and therapeutic measures, complications, outcome. Include code note, if appropriate.
   E. Your assessment and plan at this point, with brief differential diagnosis of what could be going on.
   F. Reason for transfer (pressors, arrhythmias, unstable vital signs, closer monitoring, etc.).
   G. Code status.
   H. Who has been notified (patient's physician, family members).

7

Patient and Staff Relations

. . . It's like winking in the dark, YOU know what you're doing, but make sure everyone else does, too. . . .

WORKING WITH ANCILLARY STAFF

- Give specific directions and use your judgment, but also give others a chance to make suggestions and solve problems. Effective use of ancillary staff can greatly increase your efficiency.
- A compliment for a job well done goes a long way (others are over-worked, too) and will be remembered when you need help.
- Criticize in private. Constructive feedback may be necessary and welcomed if done in a nonjudgmental manner.
- Regard ancillary staff as fellow members of the patient care team; they are often "bothering" you out of concern for the patient and not to harass you.
- Efforts to let team members know the plan can save you phone calls and increase sleep.

REFERRING A PATIENT

- When referring a patient to the ER, another physician, or admitting or transferring a patient, always be sure to make a courtesy call first.
- Pertinent information includes
  1. Who you are
  2. Patient identification information
  3. Succinct history of the problem
  4. Supporting lab data
  5. Suggestions for further evaluation
  6. Likely disposition of the patient
  7. A contact number where you or someone covering for you can be reached for questions or follow-up information

WORKING WITH DIFFICULT PATIENTS

. . . Having fun yet? . . .

- Be proactive and address potential concerns, expectations, or questions up front. Checking in with the patient at regular intervals builds rapport and can save you from multiple phone calls. Try to minimize waiting time and interruptions during meetings.
- Be as flexible and as accommodating as you can. Recognize that the patient may be tired of repeating his or her history or having a physical examination.

- Letting the patient (and loved ones) know about the management plan should be done at least once a day. Follow up with them on test results and changes in the plan, and let them know if consultants will be coming by.
- If more than one service is involved, designate someone to be the primary source of communication to avoid confusion.
- The patient's "difficult" behavior may stem from lack of control over decision making and the situation, or lack of insight into his or her medical condition. Past experiences, things the patient may have seen or read in the media, and fear may also play a role. *Active* listening, acknowledging the patient's point of view, and reassurance can go a long way.
- Acknowledge your own frustration, seek the advice of others when necessary, and always try to do what's best for the patient.

TABLE 7-1. POTENTIAL RESOURCES AND OPTIONS

Resources	Options
Nursing supervisor or manager	• Individual or joint meetings with or without loved ones (useful for any situation below)
Social worker	• Initial evaluation for nursing home, rehab, or extended care facility placement
Case coordinator	• Return to nursing home issues; durable medical equipment; insurance disputes and concerns • Home health/home infusion/hospice referrals • Transportation issues
Risk management	• For litigious patients/family members, if you have concerns about the case, or if you expect a poor outcome
Ombudsman or ethics committee	• Helpful if there are disputes between physicians or family members
Family members or loved ones	• Proceed cautiously, if there are family members who are in disagreement, try to remain neutral
Religious resources	• For issues related to death and end of life issues.
A new physician	• A new physician may be the best solution if other options have failed

TABLE 7-2. DEALING WITH DIFFICULT PROBLEMS

Problem	Suggestions	Potential Actions
Abuses of the system (i.e., narcotics)	Set boundaries, written contracts often helpful (be specific in stating the problem and plan).	• Notify all members of the team caring for the patient. • Document concisely in the chart and include on sign out.
Manipulative patients	See above. Coordinate care through one team member to maintain consistency.	See above.
Violent patients (see Chapter 17, Psychiatry section)	• *Safety first.* • Tell others you are seeing the patient. • Try to remain calm and neutral. • Always stand between the patient and the door. • Remove all potentially dangerous items that can be used against you (i.e., stethoscope).	• See above. Contact security or law enforcement officials if necessary. • Arrange to have security nearby when you see the patient.
Patients who want to leave AMA	• First, establish competence. Then, • Listen to the patient's reason(s). • Respond in a nondefensive, nonjudgmental manner. • Calmly explain the risks and consequences of leaving. • Explain the benefits of staying and the importance of completing the diagnostic/treatment plan. • Be accommodating if possible. • Enlist the help of other team/family members.	See above. • Have patient sign AMA form. • Carefully document discussion of risks and benefits in the chart. • Try to arrange discharge medications and follow-up plans. • Advise the patient to seek medical attention again if condition worsens.
Homelessness or return to abusive situations	Social work is a helpful resource.	• Refer patients to local shelters or to local shelters/safe havens. • Contact proper authorities (i.e., police, Division of Aging, Child and Family Services). • Careful, neutral documentation in the medical record.

(continued)

TABLE 7-2. DEALING WITH DIFFICULT PROBLEMS (Continued)

Problem	Suggestions	Potential Actions
Refusal of nursing home placement	• Social work, family members, and other team members can assist and discuss with patient. • Consider rehabilitation as a potential place for referral.	• Emphasize that it may be a temporary stay. • Try to arrange for close outpatient follow-up, home health services, and other family members to check in and help. • Ultimately, you may have to respect the patient's wishes.
High likelihood that patient will abuse substances again	Consider chemical dependency consult.	Inpatient or outpatient follow-up.
Concern for suicide or homicide (see Chapter 17, Psychiatry section)	Consider psychiatry consultation, assess competency.	• Document carefully in the chart. • Notify proper authorities. • Consider possible transfer to inpatient psychiatric setting. • Notify family members and loved ones.
Financial difficulties	Social worker or case coordinator can be very helpful.	• Payment and transportation arrangements can be made. • Medication samples. • Referral to free clinics and resources. • Assistance with applying for Medicaid, disability, etc.

TABLE 7-3. ADDRESSING END-OF-LIFE ISSUES

Issue	Suggestions
Code status Intubation CPR Vasopressors Cardioversion Antibiotics and other medications Nutrition (i.e., G-tubes) Phlebotomy IV lines Withdrawal of support Comfort care	Explain it in language and terms the patient and family members can understand. Remain neutral, although it is appropriate to give your opinion, especially if asked. Be very specific and clear (i.e., the exact interventions to be done or not to be done) in your discussion and **document clearly in the medical record.** **Communicate status with other team members.** Give sufficient time to consider the decision, and explain this decision can be changed. Be open and available for further discussion and questions. If patient is not able to discuss this with you, contact primary physician and family members, power of attorney.

8

Admissions

. . . When the fun begins . . .

GENERAL POINTS

1. When called with a new admission, it is critical to review old records, lab results, and old charts. However, if the patient is assessable, always eyeball the patient first and check vital signs before digging through old records. With that said, old records are invaluable. Most systems have old lab results, discharge summaries, H & Ps stored as electronic versions; use these extensively, but always confirm with your own eyes and ears.

2. After assessment of the patient and examination, admission orders should be completed as soon as possible. This will help the nursing staff and will enable you to get appropriate lab results in a timely manner. If you need stat labs, always inform the nursing staff directly. It is also helpful to inform the nurses when your orders are complete.

3. The history and physical examination should be well engrained by now. It is often helpful to dictate the H & P right after evaluating the patient. If you decide to dictate, you must ensure a signed copy of the dictation makes it into the medical record chart. A short handwritten note of the current admission problems and short assessment should also be entered in the chart while awaiting the dictated H & P. Lab results can be added manually to the dictation as an addendum.

4. If the patient has a private primary care physician, he or she should be notified as soon as possible regarding the admission, and your plan should be communicated to the private physician. Many private physicians or their covering partners like to be notified as soon as possible, regardless of the time of night.

5. In summary, remember the three pearls of an admission:
   - Assess the stability of the patient: Do this first.
   - Obtain a good H & P, even if this has already been done by another medical team.
   - Write orders as soon as possible. This makes the nurses and unit clerks happy and allows you to get the lab data you need to finish your evaluation.

ADMISSION ORDERS

Many admission diagnoses have preset clinical pathways and associated order sets (i.e., CHF, asthma). These are often helpful. Also, consider the patient's eligibility for appropriate research studies.

The mnemonic ADCVAANDISML may be useful.

A   Admit to ward/attending/house officers
D   Diagnosis
C   Condition
V   Vitals: Always include call orders (i.e., call HO for SBP >180 or <90, pulse >130 or <60, RR >30 or <10, T >38.3°C, O_2 saturation <92%)
A   Allergies
A   Activity (ad lib, bedrest with bedside commode, and so forth)
N   Nursing (strict I/O, daily weights, guaiac stools, Accuchecks, Foleys)
D   Diet (prudent diabetic, low fat/low cholesterol, renal, NPO, low salt)
I   IV (IV fluids, heplock)
S   Special (wound care, consults with social work, dietitian, PT/OT)
M   Meds [don't forget prn meds or you will be called often; if no contraindications, include acetaminophen (Tylenol), diphenhydramine (Benadryl), zolpidem (Ambien), and aluminum and magnesium hydroxide (Maalox)]
L   Laboratory (don't forget to include a.m. labs)

Don't forget DVT prophylaxis (heparin, 5000 U SQ bid; or SCDs) for every patient who is not ambulating.

ASSESSMENT/PLAN

This is the meat of your note. It is useful to separate this section by problem. The assessment should include a one-line summary of the patient's known medical problems (i.e., HTN, T2DM, CAD) and those under evaluation (i.e., fever, melena). For example, 60 y/o female with a history of hypertension, T2DM presents with new onset chest pain and fever. Include a short differential diagnosis of the current problem.

The plan should be separated by problem. Cover all problems, including stable issues, such as

1. Chest pain: No ECG changes, chest pain free now, will rule out MI, monitor on telemetry, continue beta blocker, nitrates, ASA, and ACEI. NPO for stress thallium in a.m. assuming rules out for MI.
2. Hypertension: Good control on current medical regimen.
3. T2DM: Good control with A1C of 7.2. Continue glucose checks, prudent diabetic diet. Hold PO diabetic meds while NPO. Will use insulin sliding scale while NPO.

Code status should be addressed with every patient admitted regardless of age or disease. Unexpected problems arise too often and it is better to be prepared. The patient's code status should be listed as a separate problem at the end of the list of problems.

LABORATORY RESULTS AND ORDERS

It is imperative that orders and lab tests are followed up in a timely manner. You must take personal responsibility to ensure that this is completed.

9

Daily Assessments

. . . Same bat time, same bat channel . . .

ROUNDS

. . . Round and round and round . . .

Many programs categorize rounds into prerounds, work rounds, and attending rounds.

Prerounding

Prerounding is primarily an intern's responsibility. Usually allow 30 minutes to 1 hour before rounds, depending on the number of patients on your service. The exact responsibilities should be worked out individually with your resident. It is often not necessary to physically see all of your patients before work rounds. It is customary to see those patients with an acute problem.

Probably the most important aspects are getting signouts and catching up on the overnight events (i.e., cross-cover problems). However, the following example is a good prerounding plan:

1. Get your signout from the night float or cross-cover team. You need to know of any major events that happened overnight, and this dictates how you will spend your time prerounding.
2. Check vital signs on all your patients. This can often be done on the computers. It is also helpful to check nursing notes on the computer.
3. See the patients. A quick check on your patients (2–3 minutes per patient) allows you to see how they look and if they have developed any new problems overnight. Of course, patients with more acute illness require more time.
4. Check lab results and final results of tests (i.e., CXR, Echos, etc.). Check telemetry every day on all your monitored patients.
5. For patients with private physicians, it is often helpful to discuss the plan face to face with them in the morning (i.e., try to catch them on their morning rounds). This saves you time in trying to reach them at their offices or in deciphering their progress notes.

DAILY NOTES AND EVALUATION

Interns are primarily responsible for writing daily notes on each of their patients. The SOAP format is usually used for daily notes.

S Subjective: What the patient says or what nursing staff reports. Past 24 hour events.

O Objective: Factual information, vitals, PE, lab results, lines, and tubes. Include micro, x-rays, and other studies here. Always check final official readings of tests.

A/P Assessment/Plan: This is the meat of the note. Usually catego-
rized by problem or organ system in the order of importance.
Always include fluids/electrolytes/nutrition as a problem as
well as code status in every note. In addition, the last category
or problem should be discharge planning. Include status and
goals (e.g., social work placement, home oxygen).

Active medications are often listed in a side column. This exercise can
be tedious but ensures that every medication is reviewed daily. Also include
the day number for antibiotics and other loading dose medications.

Every day, review the following items:

- Do IV lines need to be changed?
- Can IV meds be changed to PO?
- Can you discontinue the Foley?
- Can you advance the diet and increase the activity of the patient? Is
  the patient moving his or her bowels?
- PT/OT and social work: Are they involved and should they be?
  What is the status of discharge planning?
- Are all meds adjusted for renal or hepatic failure?

Daily orders should be consolidated and written as early as possible.
Every lab test and study ordered needs to be followed up. If a study
needs to be done stat or ASAP, you must notify the ward clerk and
nurse directly. It is often helpful to discuss a brief plan with the patient
and the nursing staff. This helps them to be part of the team and also
helps move things along.

DISCHARGE PLANNING

D/C planning must be addressed and readdressed constantly. Proper D/C
planning prevents large teams and reduces resident irritation. D/C planning should start on admission. Social work should be consulted on
admission if D/C needs are anticipated (assisted living, placement,
transportation). Scheduled meetings with case coordinators or social
workers are often helpful to reassess the situation and provide updates.

SIGNOUTS

Most programs have some variety of night float to help with cross-cover
overnight. Succinct but complete signouts include the following items:

- Name of patient, birth date, room number.
- List of active problems and relevant medical history (i.e., ESRD).
- Any pending studies or overnight lab tests and trends of lab results.
  Also include certain criteria to act on (i.e., transfuse 1 unit PRBC if
  Hct is <28).
- Code status: This must be specified.
- Highlight any worrisome patients and why you are concerned.
  Include suggestions on how to deal with certain problems and what
  worked earlier in the hospital course.

10 Other Notes of Importance

. . . The paper chase . . .

OFF-SERVICE NOTES

. . . Passing the buck . . .

It is your final day on the floors, you've had a grueling month, and the last thing you want to do is write another note, let alone think about writing long, drawn-out off-service notes. However, the presence of short concise off-service notes can be a life-saver to the intern coming onto the service. The essentials include the following items:

1. Date of admission
2. Major diagnoses
3. Pertinent past medical history
4. Hospital course (major interventions, events, procedures); this can be organized chronologically or by organ system, depending on the patient
5. Current medications including day number for antibiotics
6. Current pertinent PE and lab results
7. Assessment and plan

PROCEDURE NOTES

. . . See one, do one, document one . . .

These are of vital importance as part of the documentation of the hospital course and should include the following items:

1. Procedure, site of procedure
2. Indication(s)
3. Consent
4. Sterile prep used
5. Anesthesia used
6. Brief description of the procedure
7. Specimens and what they were sent for
8. Complications
9. Postprocedure disposition and pending follow-up studies (i.e., CXR post–central line placement)
10. Any fluids that you just spent your valuable time collecting should be hand delivered to the lab personally (e.g., CSF, ABG, other taps, etc.)

DEATH/EXPIRATIONS

. . . The celestial discharge . . .

Interns are called on quite frequently to pronounce a death. Certain steps must be performed.

- On arrival to the bedside, you should observe for respirations, auscultate for heart sounds, palpate for a pulse, and attempt to elicit a corneal reflex. You also need to agree on an exact time of death with the nursing staff.
- Notify the private physician and family immediately, even in the middle of the night. The family must be asked specifically about (1) autopsy, (2) anatomic gift donation, and (3) funeral home. Appropriate forms for an autopsy and anatomic gifts must be completed.
- Complete a death note in the progress note section of the chart. It should include this format: "Called by nursing to see patient regarding unresponsiveness. The patient was found to be breathless, pulseless, and without heart tones, blood pressure, and corneal reflexes. The patient was pronounced dead at 5:25 a.m. on 1/25/99. The patient's private physician and family were notified. The patient's family refused both anatomic gifts and autopsy. The funeral home will be Manchester Mortuary." The word *dead* must be used.
- The Certificate of Death must be completed. If the patient has a private physician, the death certificate will be completed by the private physician. Also, dictate a short death summary at this time.

11

Discharges

. . . Happy Trails! Come back if you have to . . .

With proper planning, discharges can be smooth for you and the patient. In today's environment, many more diseases are being managed and followed in the outpatient setting. Therefore, it is critical that the patient has follow-up, and the patient's physician is aware of any pending issues or studies. Communication with all involved parties is crucial to a successful discharge process. It also prevents many bounce backs.

DISCHARGE PROCESS/PEARLS

- Obtain social work/case coordinator assistance early in the admission. Try to anticipate issues and problems early on (e.g., transportation, home oxygen, or placement).
- Make sure the patient and his or her family are aware of possible discharge dates so they can arrange their schedules and not be caught off guard.
- Arrange for home services at least 1 day before discharge (i.e., home nursing, PT, OT, etc.).
- Criteria for home O_2:
  PaO_2 <55 mm Hg
  PaO_2 of 55–59 mm Hg with evidence of cor pulmonale or secondary polycythemia (Hct >55%)
  O_2 sat <88% on room air consistently (at rest, with exercise, or with sleep)
- Get rid of Foley catheters, telemetry monitoring, and supplemental oxygen as soon as possible. Many rehabilitation facilities require that these are not present 24 hours before discharge.
- Change antibiotics to PO the day before discharge. Avoid a.m. lab work the morning of discharge, unless absolutely necessary.
- Provide all prescription medications including three refills, excluding controlled substances. This paperwork can often be done in advance.
- Dictate the discharge summary at the time of discharge. It may seem painful at the time, but it will save you time later. It is most efficient to dictate when you are most familiar with the patient and hospital course. Take the extra 5–10 minutes to complete it now.
- The hospital course section of a well-organized discharge summary is generally organized by problem list.

DISCHARGE SUMMARY

Each institution has its own rules on discharge summaries. However, most should include the following items:

- Your name, the attending physician's name, and patient name and number
- Date of admission and discharge
- Principal and secondary diagnoses and procedures
- Chief complaint and HPI
- Hospital course
- Discharge medications, diet, and activity
- Follow-up plans
- Condition on discharge
- Copy distribution

12

Top Ten Workups

■ CHEST PAIN

. . . You may start to develop chest pain of your own. . . .
Of course, angina or MI is your first thought. However, the most important tool in identifying the cause of chest pain is a good history. The patient should be assessed immediately.

Before you hang up the phone, ask the nurse for vital signs. Initial verbal orders should include stat ECG, O_2 by NC at 2 L/min, sublingual nitroglycerin 0.4 mg, and aspirin 325 mg to bedside. Confirm IV access.

A. Major Causes of Chest Pain
Heart/vascular: Angina, MI, acute pericarditis, dissection
Lungs: Pneumonia, PE, pneumothorax
GI: Esophageal spasm, GERD, PUD, pancreatitis
Other: Costochondritis, herpes zoster

B. Things You Don't Want to Miss (Call Your Resident)
MI
Aortic dissection
PE
Pneumothorax

C. Key History
✓ Check BP, pulse, respirations, and O_2 saturations.
✓ Quickly review chart.
✓ Take a focused history including quality, duration, radiation, changes with respiration, diaphoresis, N/V.
✓ Review ECG. If cardiac etiology is suspected, give NTG SL if SBP >90. Also, make patient chew the aspirin, if not already given during the day.

D. Focused Examination

	KEY POINTS
General	How distressed or sick does the patient look?
Vitals	Hypotension is an ominous sign. Tachycardia may be from a PE or from pain. Bradycardia may be from AV block with inferior MI. Take BP in both arms.
Chest	Check for chest wall tenderness and any skin lesions. Listen for murmur, rubs, or gallops. Assess JVP.

Lungs   Assess for crackles, absent breath sounds on one
                side, friction rub.
Abdomen   Tenderness, bowel sounds.
Extremities   Edema or evidence of deep venous thrombosis. If
                dissection is suspected, examine pulses bilat-
                erally in both upper and lower extremities.

E. Laboratory Data

Check ABG if respiratory distress or low saturations are present;
serial troponins (q12h × 2), portable CXR. V̇/Q̇ scan or D-dimer
if PE is suspected; also consider lower extremity Dopplers or
contrast CT or TEE if dissection is suspected.

F. Management

➤ Cardiac: If evidence of acute MI on ECG (ST elevation of 1
mm or more in two contiguous leads or new LBBB) and history, consider reperfusion therapy; stat cardiology consult and
transfer to CCU. Consider β-blockers, nitrates, heparin, and
antiplatelet agents. Metoprolol, 5 mg IV, may be initiated and
repeated every 5 minutes for a total dose of 15 mg. Ensure the
patient is on a monitor, has IV access, has oxygen 2 L by NC,
and has received an aspirin.

➤ Angina: NTG, 0.4 mg times 3 every 5 minutes, assuming SBP
>90. Consider β-blockers, nitrates, heparin, and antiplatelet
agents. Place on telemetry.

➤ Aortic dissection: Arrange for immediate transfer to CCU/
MICU. Start nitroprusside or labetalol for BP control. Stat vas-
cular/thoracic surgery consult.

➤ Pulmonary: If PE, ensure oxygenation and administer IV heparin See Therapeutics section for dosing (Chapter 15); pain
control.

➤ Pneumothorax: Tension requires immediate needle decompression in the second intercostal space in the midclavicular line,
followed by chest tube. Other pneumothoraces involving >20%
of the lung require chest tube.

➤ GI: Antacids such as aluminum hydroxide (Maalox), 30 mL PO
prn q4–6h, famotidine (Pepcid), 20 mg PO bid, or omeprazole
(Prilosec), 20 mg PO qd. Elevate the head of the bed.

■ **ABDOMINAL PAIN**

. . . Not just from the cafeteria food . . .

What are the patient's vital signs? How severe is the pain? Is this a new problem? If vital signs are stable, inform the nurse you will be there shortly and to call you immediately if things worsen before you arrive.

A. Major Causes of Abdominal Pain

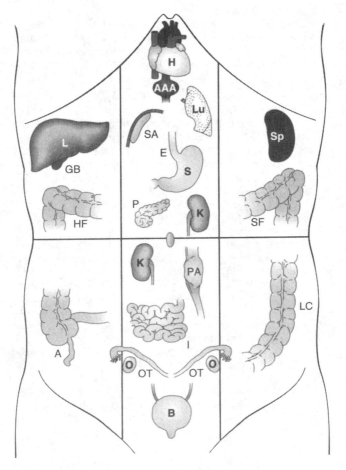

It's easiest to think of them by location:

Right upper quadrant
  L, Liver (hepatitis, abscess, perihepatitis)
  GB, Gallbladder (cholecystitis, cholangitis, choledocholithiasis)
  HF, Hepatic flexure (obstruction)

Right lower quadrant
  A, Appendix (appendicitis,* abscess)
  O, Ovary (torsion, ruptured cyst, carcinoma)
Left upper quadrant
  Sp, Spleen (rupture, infarct, abscess)
  SF, Splenic flexure (obstruction)
Left lower quadrant
  LC, Left colon (diverticulitis, ischemic colitis)
  O, Ovary (torsion, ruptured cyst, carcinoma)
Epigastrium
  H, Heart (myocardial infarction, pericarditis, aortic dissection)
  AAA, Abdominal aortic aneurysm
  Lu, Lung (pneumonia, pleurisy)
  SA, Subphrenic abscess
  E, Esophagus (gastroesophageal reflux disease)
  S, Stomach and duodenum (peptic ulcer)
  P, Pancreas (pancreatitis)
  K, Kidney (pyelonephritis, renal colic)
Hypogastrium
  K, Kidney (renal colic)
  PA, Psoas abscess
  I, Intestine (infection,* obstruction,* inflammatory bowel disease*)
  O, Ovary (torsion, ruptured cyst, carcinoma)
  OT, Ovarian tube (ectopic pregnancy, salpingitis, endometriosis)
  B, Bladder (cystitis, distended bladder)
Generalized abdominal pain
  1. See conditions marked with an *asterisk* (*).
  2. Peritonitis (any cause)
  3. Diabetic ketoacidosis
  4. Sickle cell crisis
  5. Acute intermittent porphyria
  6. Acute adrenocortical insufficiency due to steroid withdrawal

From Marshall SA, Ruedy J. *On call: principles and protocols,* 3rd ed. Philadelphia: W.B. Saunders Company, 2000.

B. Things You Don't Want to Miss (Call Your Resident)
AAA rupture
Bowel rupture or perforation
Ascending cholangitis
Acute appendicitis

C. Key History
✓ Check BP, pulse, respirations, O_2 saturations, and temperature.
✓ Quickly look at the patient and review the chart.
✓ Take a focused history, including quality, duration, radiation, changes with respiration, location, N/V (bilious versus nonbilious), last bowel movement, and any hematemesis or melena or hematochezia.

✓ Mesenteric ischemia often has pain out of proportion to examination. Consider this, especially with a history of atrial fibrillation, vascular disease, and in elderly patients.

D. Focused Examination

KEY POINTS

General	How distressed or sick does the patient look?
Vitals	Repeat now.
HEENT	Check for icterus.
Chest	Check for any skin lesions. Listen for murmur, rubs, or gallops. Assess jugular venous pulse.
Lungs	Assess for crackles, absent breath sounds on one side, friction rub.
Abdomen	Inspect bowel sounds: high pitched with SBO, absent with ileus. Percussion: tympany, shifting dullness. Palpation: guarding, rebound tenderness, Murphy's sign, psoas, and obturator signs. Assess for CVA tenderness.
Rectal	Must be performed, guaiac for occult blood.
Pelvic	If indicated by history.

E. Laboratory Data

Consider CBC, electrolytes, ABG, lactate, LFTs, amylase, lipase, β-hCG, and UA. Films to consider include flat and upright abdominal films, CXR, and ECG. Abdominal CT, ultrasound, or both may be required.

F. Management

➢ The initial goal is to determine if the patient has an acute abdomen and needs surgical evaluation and treatment. Avoid any analgesics as this may mask the pain and obscure the evaluation. An acute abdomen includes rebound tenderness or guarding and conditions such as ruptured viscus, abscess, or hemorrhage. See Acute Abdomen section (Chapter 17).

➢ Other conditions can be managed using a more detailed and leisurely approach, after the acute abdomen has been ruled out.

➢ Keep the patient NPO. Ensure IV access, and run maintenance fluids.

■ ACUTE ALTERED MENTAL STATUS

. . . Not unlike you post-call . . .

What are the patient's vital signs? What was the time course of changes? Any change in level of consciousness or any trauma? Is the patient a diabetic? Any recent narcotics or sedatives given? What was the reason for admission (i.e., alcohol)?

Initial verbal orders to consider: think of TONG (thiamine, oxygen, naloxone, and glucose). Have the nurse obtain Accucheck and oxygen saturations now.

Acute mental status changes associated with fever or decreased consciousness require that you see the patient immediately.

A. Major Causes of Acute Altered Mental Status

- Structural/CNS
  - Head trauma/subdural hematoma
  - Hydrocephalus
  - CVA/TIA
  - Dementia
  - Postictal state
  - Fecal impaction
  - Tumor or abscess
- Systemic/metabolic
  - Drugs (narcotics, benzos, and so forth), especially in elderly, even in low doses
  - Alcohol withdrawal
  - Hypoglycemia/DKA
  - Organ failure (hypoxia, hypercapnia, renal, or liver)
  - Hypertension or hypotension
  - Infection (sepsis, UTI, meningitis, especially in the setting of dementia)
  - Endocrine (thyroid, Addison's disease, increased calcium, low B_{12})

B. Things You Don't Want to Miss (Call Your Resident)

Sepsis or meningitis

Intracranial mass or increased pressure

Alcohol withdrawal (DTs)

C. Key History

✓ Check BP, pulse, respirations, O_2 saturations, temperature, and Accucheck.

✓ Quickly look at the patient and review the chart.

✓ Confirm no falls or trauma.

✓ Review chart for new meds or narcotics.

✓ Take a focused history, including onset and level of responsiveness.

D. Focused Examination

KEY POINTS

General	How distressed or sick does the patient look?
HEENT	Look for signs of trauma; pupil size, symmetry, and response to light; papilledema and nuchal rigidity.
Abdomen	Look for ascites, jaundice, and other signs of liver disease.
Neurologic	Thoroughly examine, including mental status examination, and check for asterixis.

E. Laboratory Data

Consider CBC, electrolytes, LFTs, ABG, TSH, UA, cultures, ECG, and CXR. Other studies that may be required are lumbar puncture, CT, and EEG. Never perform a lumbar puncture if you suspect a mass lesion or raised intracranial pressure, until a CT is obtained or a funduscopic examination is performed.

F. Management

➤ Management is based on findings on examination and laboratory data. If meningitis is suspected, lumbar puncture should be performed after CT or funduscopic examination. In addition, empiric antibiotics should be started stat (see Chapter 17, neurology consult section, for antibiotic choices).

➤ Alcohol withdrawal needs to be treated urgently with benzodiazepines, usually chlordiazepoxide (Librium) or lorazepam (Ativan). Thiamine should also be administered, especially before any glucose. See Chapter 13 for dosing.

■ ACUTE RENAL FAILURE

. . . Like you have time to use the bathroom . . .

What are the patient's vital signs? How much urine has been produced in the last 24 hours? In the last 8 hours? Does the patient have a Foley catheter inserted? What are the patient's recent electrolytes, especially potassium, BUN, creatinine, and bicarbonate?

If the patient does have a Foley catheter inserted, ask the nurse to flush the catheter with 30 mL NS. If the patient does not have a Foley catheter, ask the nurse to place one now. Tell the nurse you will see the patient shortly.

A. Major Causes of Oliguria

Major causes of oliguria can be broken down as follows:

- Prerenal: Volume depletion, congestive heart failure, vascular occlusion
- Renal: Glomerular, tubular/interstitial (acute tubular necrosis caused by drugs or toxins), and vascular
- Postrenal: Obstruction (BPH), clogged Foley catheter, stones

B. Things You Don't Want to Miss (Call Your Resident)

Hyperkalemia

C. Key History

✓ Check BP, pulse, respirations, O_2 saturations, and temperature.
✓ Quickly look at the patient and review the chart.
✓ Take a focused history.
✓ Determining volume status is important. Review ins and outs over the past few days. Any new medications (e.g., ACE inhibitors)?

D. Focused Examination

	KEY POINTS
General	How distressed or sick does the patient look?
Vitals	Check orthostatics and weight over the past few days.
Cardiovascular	Check for JVD, friction rub, and skin turgor.
Abdomen	Look for ascites or enlarged bladder.
Genitourinary	Check for enlarged prostate.
Extremities	Assess perfusion. Check for asterixis.

E. Laboratory Data

UA: Look for cells, casts, protein. Electrolytes, urine electrolytes, calculate FENa, urine eosinophils, ABG, and ECG. Renal ultrasound should be ordered within 24 hours to rule out hydronephrosis and evaluate the renal system.

F. Management

➢ Oliguria is generally defined as <400 mL urine per 24 hours. The minimum acceptable urine output is 30 mL/hour. If flush-

ing the Foley catheter did not help, ask the nurse to change the
Foley catheter.

➤ Initial management should be directed at treating life-threatening
electrolyte disorders and correcting volume contraction and
hypotension. Obtain diagnostic urinary studies before administering diuretics. Don't forget to adjust drug doses based on
glomerular filtration rate.

$$FENa = \frac{U[Na] \times P[Cr]}{U[Cr] \times P[Na]}$$

This equation is most useful with oliguric renal failure, but may
be helpful in nonoliguric renal failure. FENa >1% to 2% with
oliguria is almost always ATN, but can be prerenal with diuretics. FENa <1% with oliguria is generally prerenal: volume
depletion, severe CHF, or nephrotic syndrome, NSAID or dye
toxicity, sepsis, cyclosporine toxicity, acute GN, and hepatorenal
syndrome. Also calculate FE urea in nonoliguric renal failure.

➤ Hyperkalemia, CHF, severe acidemia, and pericarditis require
immediate attention. Obtain recent electrolytes and a stat potassium.

➤ If hyperkalemia suspected, order an ECG. A stat renal consult
is required if the patient needs urgent dialysis. Indications for
urgent dialysis include
1. Hyperkalemia (unable to reduce medically)
2. Volume overload
3. Acidemia pH <7.2
4. Uremic encephalopathy
5. Uremic pericarditis
Treatment of hyperkalemia is covered in Chapter 13.

➤ **Prerenal causes** can be initially managed with a small volume
challenge, such as 250–500 mL NS bolus depending on the cardiovascular status of the patient. This can be followed by NS at
a set rate. Specific criteria should be given to the nursing staff
(i.e., call HO if urine output is <30 mL/hr). Alternatively, if
congestive heart failure is suspected, the patient may need
diuresis. Escalating doses of furosemide (Lasix) can be used
and the urine output can be assessed. With a fluid challenge, the
creatinine level often trends down by the next morning if the
cause is prerenal.

➤ **Postrenal causes** can be potentially managed by placing a
Foley catheter. If immediate flow is obtained, urethral obstruction is likely.

➤ For contrast-induced ARF prophylaxis, normovolemia is essential. Use $\frac{1}{2}$ NS at 75 mL/hour for 12 hours.

■ HEADACHE

... Like your head isn't pounding by now ...

What are the patient's vital signs? How severe is the headache? Has there been a change in consciousness? Has the patient had similar headaches in the past; if so, what relieves them?

If the headache is severe and acute or associated with N/V, changes in vision, fever, or decreased consciousness, the patient should be seen immediately. Otherwise, inform the nurse you will see the patient shortly.

A. Major Causes of Headache

Tension

Vascular (migraine, subarachnoid hemorrhage)

Cluster

Drugs

Temporal arteritis

Infectious (meningitis, sinusitis)

Trauma

CVA and hypertension

Mass lesions

B. Things You Don't Want to Miss (Call Your Resident)

Meningitis

Subarachnoid hemorrhage

Mass lesion associated with herniation

C. Key History

✓ Check BP, pulse, respirations, O_2 saturations, and temperature.

✓ Quickly look at the patient and review the chart.

✓ A detailed, well-focused history is the best method for evaluating a headache. Most are tension or migraine type, but more serious conditions need to be ruled out.

D. Focused Examination

KEY POINTS

General	How distressed or sick does the patient look?
HEENT	Look for signs of trauma, pupil size, symmetry, response to light, papilledema, nuchal rigidity, temporal artery tenderness, and sinus tenderness.
Neurologic	Thorough examination, including mental status.

E. Laboratory Data

Consider CBC and ESR if temporal arteritis suspected. Head CT should be considered if

1. A chronic headache pattern has changed or new severe headache occurs
2. In a patient older than 50 years
3. Focal findings on neurologic examination.

If meningitis is suspected, lumbar puncture should be performed. If there is no papilledema and no focal neurologic findings, lumbar puncture should not be delayed for a CT scan, especially if the CT cannot be done within 1 hour.

F. Management

➤ The initial goal is to exclude the serious life-threatening conditions mentioned previously. After such conditions have been excluded, management can focus on symptomatic relief.

➤ Tension headaches and mild migraines can be treated with acetaminophen (Tylenol), 650 mg PO q6h prn, ibuprofen (Motrin), 200–600 mg PO q6–8h, sumatriptan (Imitrex), 25 mg PO, can repeat 25–100 mg q2h for maximum of 200–300 mg/day.

➤ Severe migraines may require a narcotic such as meperidine or codeine. Sumatriptan or ergotamine are usually most effective in the prodromal stage. These agents are contraindicated in patients with angina, uncontrolled hypertension, hemiplegia, or basilar artery migraine.

■ HYPOTENSION AND HYPERTENSION

. . . Too high, too low, uh oh . . .

Hypotension

What are the patient's vital signs? Is the patient conscious, confused, or disoriented? What has the patient's blood pressure been? What was the reason for admission?

If impending or established shock is suspected, ensure IV access and have the patient placed in Trendelenburg's position (head of bed down). Hypotension requires that you see the patient immediately.

A. Major Causes of Hypotension

Cardiogenic (rate or pump problem)
Hypovolemic
Septic shock
Anaphylaxis

B. Things You Don't Want to Miss (Call Your Resident)

Shock, which is evidence of inadequate perfusion. This is best assessed by looking at end organs: brain (mental status), heart (chest pain), and kidneys (urine output). Shock is a clinical diagnosis defined as a systolic BP <90, with evidence of inadequate tissue perfusion.

C. Key History

✓ Check BP, pulse, respirations, O_2 saturations, and temperature.
✓ Quickly look at the patient and review chart. Get an ECG.

D. Focused Examination

	KEY POINTS
General	How distressed or sick does the patient look?
Vitals	Repeat now. Elevated temperature and hypotension suggest sepsis.
Neurologic	Mentation.
Cardiovascular	Heart rate, JVP, skin temperature, and color. Capillary refill.
Lungs	Listen for crackles. Breath sounds on both sides.
GI	Any evidence of blood loss?

E. Laboratory Data

Consider troponins, ECG, ABG, CBC, electrolytes, or CXR.

F. Management

➤ Examine the ECG and take the pulse yourself. Check BP in both arms. A compensatory sinus tachycardia is an expected appropriate response to hypotension. However, check the ECG to ensure that the patient does not have atrial fibrillation, SVT, or ventricular tachycardia, which may cause hypotension because of decreased diastolic filling. Bradycardia may be seen in autonomic dysfunction or heart block.

> Most causes of shock require fluids to normalize the intravascular volume. Use normal saline or lactated Ringer's. The exception is cardiogenic shock, which may require preload reduction and transfer to a unit.

> Hypovolemic, anaphylactic, and septic shock require fluids. Use small boluses (e.g., 500 mL). If no response, repeat bolus or leave fluids open.

> Anaphylactic shock requires epinephrine, 0.3 mg IV immediately and repeated every 10–15 minutes as required. Hydrocortisone, 250 mg IV, and diphenhydramine (Benadryl), 25 mg IV, should also be administered.

> In septic shock, IV fluids and antibiotics can resolve the shock. However, continuing hypotension requires ICU admission for vasopressors.

> Cardiogenic shock can be the result of an acute MI or worsening CHF. However, other causes of hypotension and elevated JVP include acute cardiac tamponade, PE, and tension pneumothorax. These always need to be considered.

Hypertension

... Feel YOUR blood pressure rising? ...

What are the patient's vital signs? What has the patient's blood pressure been? What is the reason for admission? What BP medications has the patient been taking? Does the patient have signs of hypertensive emergency?

The rate of rise of the BP and the setting in which the high BP is occurring are more important than the level of BP itself. Elevated blood pressure alone, in the absence of symptoms or new or progressive target organ damage, rarely requires emergent therapy.

Hypertensive emergencies require that you see the patient immediately. Make sure the patient has an IV and order an ECG. Inform the nurse that you will arrive shortly.

A. Hypertensive Emergencies
Encephalopathy
Intracranial hemorrhage
Unstable angina or MI
Acute left ventricular failure with pulmonary edema
Aortic dissection
Eclampsia

Hypertensive Urgencies
Upper levels of stage 3 hypertension (180/110)
Optic disc edema
Severe perioperative hypertension

B. Things You Don't Want to Miss (Call Your Resident)
Hypertensive emergencies

C. Key History
✓ Check BP, pulse, respirations, O_2 saturations, and temperature.
✓ Quickly look at the patient and review the chart. Get an ECG.

D. Focused Examination

	KEY POINTS
General	How distressed or sick does the patient look?
Vitals	Repeat BP now in both arms.
Neurologic	Mentation, confusion, delirium.
HEENT	Fundi for papilledema and hypertensive changes.
Cardiovascular	Heart rate, jugular venous pulse, color. Capillary refill.
Lungs	Listen for crackles, breath sounds on both sides.

E. Laboratory Data
Consider troponins, ECG, ABG, CBC, electrolytes, or CXR.

F. Management
➤ Treat the patient, not the BP reading. Acute lowering of BP of asymptomatic patients with long-standing hypertension can be dangerous.

➤ Hypertensive emergencies require an ICU setting. Goal is to reduce the MAP by no more than 25% in the first 2 hours. IV hydralazine, nitroprusside, labetalol, or enalapril are often used. While arranging transfer to the ICU, certain wards allow medications to be started. Consider IV nitroglycerin for hypertension associated with MI or pulmonary edema. Nitroprusside is useful in aortic dissection, but should not be used without a β-blocker. Nitroprusside is also used with encephalopathy, but often requires intraarterial blood pressure monitoring.

➤ Hypertensive urgencies can usually be managed with oral doses with the goal of reducing BP over 24–48 hours. Examples include captopril, 25 mg, clonidine, 0.1 mg, or labetalol, 200–400 mg. These can be repeated or titrated every 2–4 hours. Close follow-up is essential.

■ COMMON ARRHYTHMIAS

. . . Too fast, too slow, or too irregular . . .
What are the patient's vital signs, including temperature? Any chest pain or shortness of breath?

Order a stat ECG. Patients with chest pain, shortness of breath, or hypotension need to be seen immediately.

A. Major Causes of Rapid Heart Rate and Slow Rates
- Rapid rates
    Regular: sinus tachycardia, SVT, ventricular tachycardia, atrial flutter
    Irregular: atrial fibrillation, multifocal atrial tachycardia
- Slow rates
    Drugs (β-blockers, CCB, digoxin)
    Sick sinus, MI
    AV block

B. Things You Don't Want to Miss (Call Your Resident)
Ventricular tachycardia
Hypotension or angina or MI

C. Key History
✓ Check BP, pulse, respirations, O_2 saturations, and temperature.
✓ Quick look at patient and quick review of chart. Get an ECG.

D. Focused Examination

	KEY POINTS
General	How distressed or sick does the patient look?
Vitals	Repeat now.
Neurologic	Mentation.
Cardiovascular	Heart rate, jugular venous pulse, skin temperature and color, capillary refill.
Lungs	Listen for crackles and breath sounds on both sides.

E. Laboratory Data
Consider troponins, ECG, ABG, CBC, electrolytes, or CXR.

F. Management
➤ Transfer to high-risk cardiology or telemetry floor.
➤ If patient is hypotensive and has atrial fibrillation with RVR, SVT, or ventricular tachycardia, emergency cardioversion may be required.
➤ In general, if the patient is unstable with serious signs or symptoms, a ventricular rate greater than 150, or both, you should prepare for immediate cardioversion. The patient may require sedation—call your resident. Serious signs and symptoms per ACLS protocol include chest pain, shortness of breath,

decreased level of consciousness, hypotension and shock, congestive heart failure, and acute MI. Refer to the proper ACLS algorithm at this point (see Chapter 2) and call your resident.

➤ Always complete the ABCs first and ensure O_2, and IV access and attach monitor.

➤ Atrial fibrillation with rapid rate but without evidence of hemodynamic compromise can be rate controlled with diltiazem or digoxin. See ECG section (Chapter 16) for dosing.

➤ SVT without evidence of hemodynamic compromise can sometimes be broken with Valsalva's maneuver, carotid sinus (one side at a time and always listen for bruits first), or both. If still in SVT, try adenosine, 6 mg rapid IV push, followed by 12 mg if no success. If the complex width is narrow with stable BP, verapamil, 2.5–5.0 mg, or diltiazem, 10 mg IV, can be used. If wide complex, manage as stable VT.

➤ For ventricular tachycardia, if pulseless or without BP, manage as ventricular fibrillation. If ventricular tachycardia with serious signs or symptoms, consider immediate synchronized cardioversion. If stable, start lidocaine, 1 mg/kg IV push, and follow the ACLS protocol.

■ FEVER

. . . Of known or unknown origin . . .
What are the patient's vital signs? What was the reason for admission?
Is this a new finding? Any associated symptoms (i.e., cough, headache,
change in mental status, N/V, and so forth)? Any antipyretics or current
antibiotics? Any recent surgeries (think of postoperative fever)?

Order blood and urine cultures. Patients with meningitis symptoms
or hypotension need to be seen immediately.

A. Major Causes of Fever

- Infections: Best to think of by site—lung, urine, IV sites, blood, CNS, abdomen and pelvis, GI. Consider immunocompetent status.
- Drug-induced fever: Many drugs have been implicated.
- Neoplasms
- Connective tissue diseases
- Pulmonary embolism/deep venous thrombosis
- Fever of unknown origin

B. Things You Don't Want To Miss

Meningitis
Septic shock

C. Key History

✓ Check BP, pulse, respirations, O_2 saturations, and temperature.
✓ Quickly look at the patient and review the chart.

D. Focused Examination

	KEY POINTS
General	How distressed or sick does the patient look?
Vitals	Repeat now. Tachycardia is an expected finding with fever. Recheck blood pressure.
Neurologic	Mentation, photophobia, neck stiffness, Brudzinski's or Kernig's signs.
Cardiovascular	Heart rate, jugular venous pulse, skin temperature and color. Any new murmurs? Capillary refill.
Lungs	Listen for crackles and breath sounds on both sides.
Abdomen	Assess for RUQ tenderness and bowel sounds.
Extremities	Check IV sites and signs of deep venous thrombosis or joint effusions.

E. Laboratory Data

Consider CBC, blood cultures (two sets at different sites), CMP,
UA and culture, sputum culture and Gram's stain, CXR. LP if
meningitis is suspected. Consider *Clostridium difficile* stool
cultures.

F. Management

➤ Rule out hemodynamic instability. Review medications and obtain cultures. Give antipyretics and acetaminophen, 650 mg PO or PR. Ensure IV access and consider maintenance fluids including insensible losses.

➤ Consider antibiotics. If the patient is hemodynamically stable, immunocompetent, not toxic appearing, with no clear source of infection, it may be prudent to withhold antibiotics and recheck cultures.

➤ Patients with fever and hypotension require broad-spectrum antibiotics and IV fluids or pressors to manage the hypotension. Septic shock is an emergency. (Please refer to Hypotension Management earlier in this chapter.)

➤ Patients with fever and neutropenia require broad-spectrum antibiotics and often need double β-lactam coverage. (Refer to the *Sanford Manual* for choices.)

➤ Patients with fever and meningitis symptoms require antibiotics immediately. Do not wait for the LP kit. Give the antibiotics, then approach the LP.

➤ Consider changing or removing Foley catheters and any indwelling IV sites.

■ SHORTNESS OF BREATH

. . . You were in good physical shape . . .)

What are the patient's vital signs, including temperature? When was the onset of SOB and what is the reason for admission? Does the patient have COPD or is the patient getting oxygen?

Order oxygen, albuterol, or ipratropium (Atrovent) nebulizer and an ABG kit to the bedside. Patients with SOB need to be seen immediately.

A. Major Causes of Shortness of Breath
Pulmonary: Asthma and COPD
Cardiovascular: CHF and pulmonary embolism
Others: Pneumothorax, tamponade, obstruction, and anxiety

B. Things You Don't Want to Miss (Call Your Resident)
Inadequate tissue oxygenation (i.e., hypoxia)

C. Key History
✓ Check BP, pulse, respirations, O_2 saturations, and temperature.
✓ Quickly look at the patient and review the chart. Get an ECG and ABG if the patient looks sick.

D. Focused Examination
KEY POINTS

General	How distressed or sick does the patient look?
Vitals	Repeat now. Check for a pulsus paradoxus.
Neurologic	Mentation and check for central cyanosis.
Cardiovascular	Heart rate, jugular venous pulse, skin temperature and color, capillary refill.
Lungs	Listen for crackles and breath sounds on both sides.

E. Laboratory Data
Consider ABG, ECG, troponins, CBC, D-dimer, $\dot{V}/\dot{Q}$ scan, and CXR.

F. Management
➤ Order empiric oxygen to keep saturations >92%. Be cautious if the patient has COPD and is a retainer of CO_2. Remember that the O_2 saturation tells you nothing about pH or P_{CO_2}.
➤ For pulmonary embolism, look for predisposing causes: the classic ECG is S_1, Q_3, and T_3. Often the patient is tachycardic and tachypneic and has a sudden onset of SOB. If suspicion is high, consider starting heparin or LMWH. Ensure that the patient has no history of bleeding disorders, PUD, recent CVA, or surgery. Obtain a $\dot{V}/\dot{Q}$ scan or spiral CT. Also, consider lower extremity Dopplers and D-dimer.
➤ For CHF, is the patient volume overloaded? Raise the head of the patient's bed. Administer Lasix, 20–40 mg IV, and albuterol nebulizer. Consider morphine or nitroglycerin. Assess for adequate diuresis.
➤ For asthma and COPD, administer albuterol and Atrovent nebulizer, q2–4h until stable. Consider IV corticosteroids, methylprednisolone (Solu-Medrol), 60 mg IV q6h, and antibiotics if needed.
➤ Acute respiratory failure is generally defined by ABG of P_{O_2} <50 or P_{CO_2} >50 with a pH <7.30 while on room air. Ensure that the patient hasn't received narcotics recently. If so, consider naloxone, 0.2 mg IV. Acute respiratory acidosis with a pH <7.20 usually requires mechanical ventilation.

■ GASTROINTESTINAL BLEEDING

. . . Ahh, the smell of melena . . .

What are the patient's vital signs? When was the onset of bleeding and what is the reason for admission? Is the bleeding upper (coffee ground emesis, melena) or lower (hematochezia)? How much blood has been lost?

Confirm that the patient has IV access and recent CBC. Type and cross-match blood. If the patient is tachycardic or hypotensive, see the patient immediately.

A. Major Causes of Gastrointestinal Bleeding

- Upper: Esophageal varices, Mallory-Weiss tear, peptic ulcer, esophagitis, neoplasm, aortoenteric fistula (history of AAA repair)
- Lower: Diverticulosis, angiodysplasia, neoplasm, IBD, infectious colitis, anorectal disease (hemorrhoids, fissures)

B. Things You Don't Want to Miss (Call Your Resident)

GI bleeding leading to hypovolemic shock.

C. Key History

✓ Check BP, pulse, respirations, O_2 saturations, and temperature. Orthostatic BP.
✓ Quickly look at the patient and review the chart.

D. Focused Examination

	KEY POINTS
General	How distressed or sick does the patient look?
Vitals	Repeat now.
Neurologic	Mentation.
Cardiovascular	Heart rate, jugular venous pulse, skin temperature and color, capillary refill.

E. Laboratory Data

Consider ECG, CBC, coags, and CMP.

F. Management

➤ Consider whether special blood products are required based on comorbidities (e.g., irradiated, washed RBCs). Also consider whether the patient needs premedication with Tylenol/Benadryl based on prior transfusions.
➤ Insert two large-bore IVs (16–18 gauge), type and cross PRBCs. It can take up to 8 hours for CBC to equilibrate, so initial Hct may be falsely elevated. In absence of renal disease, high BUN suggests GI bleeding. Check coags and platelets to exclude bleeding disorders. Is the patient receiving anticoagulants? If so, consider reversal with vitamin K or FFP.
➤ Replenish the intravascular volume by giving IV fluids (normal saline), especially while awaiting blood products. Keep the patient NPO.

➤ For upper GI bleeding, insert a nasogastric tube to assess if active bleeding is present. Suppress acid with omeprazole, 40 mg PO bid. GI consult for endoscopy. If bleeding has stopped and the patient is hemodynamically stable, elective endoscopy can be performed within the next 24 hours. Otherwise, urgent endoscopy may be required.

➤ Varices should be treated as upper GI bleeding, but also consider octreotide, 50 μg bolus, then 50 μg/hour and correct coagulation deficits.

➤ For lower GI bleeding, correct fluid status. If hemodynamically stable, obtain GI consult for colonoscopy. If unstable, an urgent tagged RBC scan should be scheduled. Also, consider arteriography.

➤ For abnormal coags, FFP and platelets may be required.

➤ Surgery consult/indications include the following:
  1. Aortoenteric fistula
  2. Uncontrollable or recurrent bleeding
  3. Bleeding episode requiring transfusion of more than 6 units PRBCs
  4. Visible naked vessel seen in peptic ulcer by endoscopy

13 Common Calls and Complaints

. . . Call me again. Go ahead, make my day . . .

ALCOHOL WITHDRAWAL

Alcohol withdrawal can be a problem both medically and behaviorally. The biggest danger is delirium tremens (DTs), which has up to a 15% mortality rate and requires close monitoring. Watch for DT symptoms of confusion, tachycardia, dilated pupils, and diaphoresis, usually 2 to 7 days after the last drink, although other symptoms can occur before then. DTs should be managed with sedatives promptly. IV fluids and electrolyte repletion are also helpful. If the patient is not in imminent danger, but is symptomatic, consider management with the following steps until substance abuse treatment can be arranged.

1. Place the patient in an environment where the patient is not endangering him- or herself or others.
2. Consider lorazepam (Ativan), 0.5–1.0 mg PO/IV/IM q6–8h (scheduled or prn), for symptoms of withdrawal. Use sitter or restraints as necessary.
3. Another alternative is chlordiazepoxide (Librium), 100 mg PO qid, for acute management; taper dose over several days.
4. Thiamine, 100 mg PO/IV/IM qd, and folate, 1 mg PO qd, can be given as preventive measures.
5. Strongly encourage the patient to seek substance abuse treatment and counseling. Social workers can assist with suggestions, and chemical dependency consultation can also be arranged for inpatient and outpatient detoxification.

BLEEDING AT LINE SITES AND AFTER PROCEDURES

Bleeding at central line sites is a common problem. Consider oozing, coagulation disorders, antiplatelet and anticoagulation drugs as causes of bleeding. Confirm that bleeding does not extend into the soft tissues of the neck, causing upper airway obstruction. Under sterile conditions, remove the dressing and apply continuous pressure to the entry site for 15 minutes. If the bleeding has stopped, clean the site and apply occlusive dressing. If bleeding has not stopped, suspect a coagulation disorder. A single suture may help provide hemostasis.

When bleeding occurs after cardiac catheterization, the cardiology fellow should be notified immediately. Initial management can be occlusive pressure and sandbag. Consider obtaining a CBC if there is protracted bleeding.

CONSTIPATION

Constipation is one of the most common complaints or calls of hospitalized patients and is something you can usually handle over the telephone. Make sure the patient isn't having N/V, abdominal pain, or fecal impaction. If these are suspected, you must see the patient. Otherwise, consider the following agents:

1. Docusate (Colace), 100 mg PO bid (stool softener). Consider giving as prevention to any patient on narcotics or bedridden patients. Usually doesn't produce the necessary effect desired unless used prophylactically.
2. Docusate/casanthranol (Peri-Colace), 1–2 tablets PO qhs prn (softener plus stimulant).
3. Bisacodyl (Dulcolax), 10 mg PO/PR prn (stimulant).
4. Consider enemas if oral agents have not been effective. Fleet or tap water enemas can be used.
5. Lactulose, 30 cc PO q4–6h, until bowel movement . . . as a last resort.

COUGH

Cough is one of the most irritating symptoms both for the patient and the house officer. Make sure the patient isn't having massive hemoptysis (defined as >600 mL over 48 hours or enough to impair gas exchange) and try to diagnose the underlying cause. Symptomatically, consider the following steps:

1. Guaifenesin/dextromethorphan or codeine (Robitussin DM or AC), 10 mL PO q4h prn
2. Codeine, 10–20 mg PO q4–6h prn
3. Benzonatate capsules (Tessalon Perles), 100 mg PO tid

DIARRHEA

Diarrhea is defined as increasing frequency and/or increasing fluidity of stools.
- Acute diarrhea is frequently self-limited.
- Determine extent of associated symptoms (N/V, blood in stools, abdominal pain).
- Consider obtaining CBC, electrolytes, and stool sample (WBCs, culture and sensitivity, ova and parasites). Also consider *Clostridium difficile* toxin assay if recent antibiotic use.
- Don't forget the possibility of ischemic colitis and fecal impaction with overflow incontinence.
- Be careful about patients on corticosteroids with minimal abdominal symptoms having an intraabdominal process.
- Consider the following items:
  1. NPO with IV hydration.
  2. Consider correcting electrolytes.

3. Discontinue possible causes including laxatives, antibiotics, antacids with magnesium.
4. Loperamide, 4 mg initially, and then 2 mg PO with each loose bowel movement. Be cautious with infectious colitis.
5. Bismuth subsalicylate (Pepto-Bismol), 30 mL PO q6h.

FALLS

1. Ask nursing for a bedside glucose test and vital signs.
2. Go see the patient.
3. Find out from the patient what occurred and where the patient is having pain. Also talk with witnesses.
4. Perform a neurologic examination, including the level of consciousness and head examination, and look for hematomas.
5. If you have any concerns about head trauma or note a change in mental status, check a stat head CT without contrast to rule out a bleed.
6. Check recent lab results and ECG/telemetry. Consider checking films for possible trauma.
7. Look at the medication list for possible contributing factors (sedatives, antihypertensives, hypoglycemic agents).
8. Clearly document what occurred in the patient's chart.

HYPERGLYCEMIA AND HYPOGLYCEMIA

Hyperglycemia

The severity should be determined by the glucose level and patient's symptoms. Confirm that the patient is not receiving IV fluids containing glucose. Most type 2 diabetics should be on a scheduled sliding scale insulin dose. A conservative scale is as follows, with Accuchecks qid:

GLUCOSE	REGULAR INSULIN SQ
60–200	0 U
201–250	2 U
251–300	4 U
301–350	6 U
351–400	8 U
>400	10 U and call house officer
<60	1 Amp D50 IV and call house officer. If taking PO, can give PO juice/crackers, etc.

- Severe hyperglycemia with DKA is a medical emergency and is not covered here.
- All type 1 diabetics require scheduled dosages of insulin.

Hypoglycemia

Any symptomatic patient with hypoglycemia should be treated. With mild hypoglycemia, oral sweetened juices can be given. With increasing severity, D50 should be given IV (1 Amp). If IV access is unavailable with severe hypoglycemia, glucagon, 1.0 mg SQ or IM, can be given. Review the patient's medications for oral hypoglycemics. If ongoing hypoglycemia occurs or the patient is NPO, start a maintenance D5W infusion at 75–100 mL/hr.

HOLDING MEDICATIONS FOR MORNING TESTS

Many tests require that patients are NPO. Always consider making patient's NPO after midnight if there is potential for testing the following day. Most orders are written NPO after midnight except medications. Certain tests (cardiac stress tests) require that you also hold β-blockers and calcium channel blockers the morning of the test. Hold Metformin 24 hours prior to studies involving IV iodinated contrast. If the test is canceled, make sure to restart the diet. For specific recommendations, please refer to Preparation for Radiologic and Endoscopic Procedures (see Chapter 16).

INSOMNIA

Insomnia is a common problem in the hospital. The patient's mental status must be considered before administering medications. Make sure delirium and dementia aren't present as well as pain that may be keeping the patient awake.

Otherwise, consider use of the following agents:

1. Antihistamines such as diphenhydramine, 25 mg PO qhs prn. Be conscious of anticholinergic side effects, especially in the elderly.
2. Zolpidem (Ambien), 5–10 mg PO qhs prn.
3. Benzodiazepines such as Restoril, 15–30 mg PO qhs prn.

LACK OF INTRAVENOUS ACCESS

Determine if IV access is necessary (i.e., essential IV medications such as antibiotics, transfusions, etc.).

Consider if IV medications can be given orally.

If access is necessary, see the patient and attempt peripheral line placement. If not successful, call IV therapy for assistance. Then consider other types of access such as PICC lines. If these are not options, consider central venous access. Please refer to Guide to Procedures (see Chapter 18).

NAUSEA AND VOMITING

Nausea and vomiting are always a symptom of an underlying etiology (*like having eaten hospital food on- or post-call*). While working up the underlying cause and eliminating life-threatening etiologies, consider using the following agents:

1. Prochlorperazine (Compazine), 5–10 mg IV/PO/IM q4–6h prn (also in suppository form, 25 mg bid)
2. Metoclopramide (Reglan), 10 mg PO/IV q6h prn
3. Trimethobenzamide (Tigan), 250 mg PO q6–8h prn

PRURITUS

While identifying the underlying cause, consider the use of the following agents:

1. Diphenhydramine (Benadryl), 25–50 mg PO q6–8h prn (or other antihistamine)
2. Hydroxyzine (Atarax, Vistaril), 25 mg PO q6–8h prn
3. Sarna lotion

RASH

First, make sure that this is not an *anaphylactic* reaction.

Specifically look for an urticarial rash with associated SOB, wheezing, laryngeal edema, and hypotension.

If these symptoms are present, consider the following items:

1. Large-bore (16 gauge) access for IV fluids
2. Epinephrine, 0.5 mg (1:1,000 solution) IV or SQ
3. Benadryl, 50 mg IV or 50–100 mg IM
4. Hydrocortisone, 250 mg IV
5. Intubation if the airway is compromised.

The most common cause of rashes in-house is a *drug reaction.*

- Hold medication that may be the cause if this is not an essential medication.
- Benadryl, 25–50 mg PO q6–8h p.m.; Atarax, 25 mg PO q6–8h p.m.; Allegra, 180 mg PO qd; or Claritin, 10 mg PO qd if itching is present.
- Corticosteroid creams or PO steroids, if severe.
- Consider dermatology consult or allergy consult (for desensitization) in a.m. (see Chapter 17).

SUNDOWNING

This is a common call overnight. The patient can present with confusion, disorientation, or combativeness in the evening hours. Things to consider:

1. Identify and treat any underlying conditions that could be contributing.
2. Minimize sedation. If absolutely necessary, haloperidol (Haldol), 0.25 mg PO/IM qd; increase to 1–5 mg as needed.
3. Provide frequent reorientation; family members can be helpful.
4. Maintain a quiet structured environment to help calm down the patient.

TRANSFUSION REACTIONS

1. If an acute hemolytic reaction is suspected, follow these steps:
   A. Immediately stop the transfusion and send bags and patient's blood sample to the laboratory for testing, including cross-match, Coombs' test, CBC, DIC panel, total bilirubin, and BMP.
   B. Rehydrate with intravascular fluid.
   C. Closely monitor renal function.
   D. Keep urine output >100 mL/hr.
2. If severe, nonhemolytic reaction is suspected (including anaphylactic symptoms, wheezing, respiratory distress, temperature >40°C)
   - D/C transfusion and send bag and line for repeat cross-match.
   - Consider diphenhydramine, 25–50 mg PO/IV.
   - Consider hydrocortisone, 250 mg IV.
   - Consider epinephrine, 0.5–1.0 mL (1:1,000) IM.
3. Volume overload
   - Decrease rate of transfusion.
   - Consider furosemide, 20–40 mg IV.
4. Fever <40°C.
   - Slow down rate of transfusion.
   - Acetaminophen, 650 mg PO.
   - Continue monitoring.

14 Pain Control

. . . As if anything could control YOUR pain . . .

GENERAL POINTS

- Treating undiagnosed pain can be perilous: always have a plan under way to diagnose the source and type of pain you are treating.
- Pain is often an undertreated symptom; once a diagnosis is made, the patient should have enough pain medications to keep him or her comfortable.
- Scheduled pain medications at appropriate doses are a viable alternative to try before switching or adding medications.
- Standing pain medication orders (can write: "patient can refuse" or "for breakthrough pain") can minimize phone calls and interrupted sleep. You will want to be notified, though, if the patient's pain or symptoms(s) persist or worsen as this may signal a change in the patient's condition.
- Consider getting an anesthesia or pain consult for other options in persistent, severe, uncontrolled pain.
- Before prescribing pain medications, always consider comorbidities, allergies, drug–drug interactions, and potential side effects.
- Trust your instincts. If you think a patient is manipulative and drug-seeking, set your boundaries and stick with them. Questions to ask:
  1. Does the patient only ask for pain medications when you are in the room?
  2. Do others observe different behaviors when you leave the room?
  3. Is the patient talking or resting comfortably?
  4. Is the patient allergic to every pain medication except the one he or she is requesting?

TABLE 14-1. SELECTED AGENTS IN THE THREE-STEP ANALGESIC LADDER

Agent	Oral	Parenteral
STEP 1 MILD PAIN: NONOPIOID		
Acetaminophen	650 mg q4–6h PRN or 1,000 mg q6h PRN	—
Aspirin	650 mg q4–6h PRN or 1,000 mg q6h PRN	—
Ibuprofen	400–800 mg q6–8h PRN	—
Gabapentin (for neuro-pathic pain)	Start 300 mg qhs	—
STEP 2 MODERATE PAIN: WEAK OPIOID (± nonopioid)		
Tylenol #3 (codeine 30 mg/ acetaminophen 300 mg)	1–2 tablets PO q4h PRN	—
Percocet (oxycodone 5 mg/ acetaminophen 325 mg)	1–2 tablets q4–6h PRN	—
Oxycodone	5 mg q4–6h	—
Tramadol	50–100 mg q4–6h (maxi-mum, 400 mg/day)	—
STEP 3 SEVERE PAIN: STRONG OPIOID (± nonopioid)		
Morphine	10–30 mg q3–4h (around the clock or intermittent dosing)	0.1–0.2 mg/kg (up to 15 mg) q4h
Morphine (controlled release)	Can start 30 mg q8–12h and increase PRN to 90–120 mg q12h	—
Fentanyl[a]	—	0.1 mg q1–3h
Hydromorphone	2–4 mg q4–6h	1–4 mg q4–6h
Levorphanol	2 mg q6–8h	2 mg q6–8h
Oxymorphone	—	1 mg q3–4h
Morphine PCA pump	1 mg/hr basal rate, 1 mg q15 minute lockout, but individualize per patient	Individualize per patient

[a]Transdermal fentanyl: 100 µg/hr = 315–404 mg/day of oral morphine and 53–67 mg/day of IM morphine.
All medications in PO form unless otherwise denoted.

Consider giving Peri-Colace or its equivalent with sustained narcotic use.

Adapted from Jacox et al., 1994, and World Health Organization, 1996.

15 Therapeutic Considerations

Antibiotics and anticoagulation are two of the most common therapeutics in the hospital setting.

ANTIBIOTICS

. . . Dose, trough, peak—just a therapeutic level I seek . . .

General Points

Three main issues must be addressed when selecting antibiotics:

1. Expected pathogen and patient demographics (i.e., nosocomial, immunocompromised)
2. Patient allergies
3. Renal and hepatic function

See *The Sanford Guide to Antimicrobial Therapy* for specific choices by site as well as renal dose adjustments and drug–drug interactions.

Some Specifics on Commonly Used Antibiotics

Vancomycin

Use in severe gram-positive infections or MRSA/ORSA. The dose is based on body weight, whereas the dosing interval is based on creatinine clearance.

Body Weight (kg)	Dose (mg)
<45	500
45–60	750
61–90	1,000
>90	1,250–1,500

CrCl (mL/min)	Interval
>60	12 hours
35–60	24 hours
15–34	48 hours
<15	Random dosing

- Drug levels are not recommended for patients receiving a short course of therapy (<5 days).
- Periodic trough levels (every week) are recommended in patients receiving longer courses of therapy to ensure concentrations are adequate. Trough levels should be obtained approximately 30 minutes before the next dose. Therapeutic trough levels range from 5–15 mg/L. Peak levels are generally not of benefit.
- Serum creatinine should be monitored weekly.

Aminoglycosides

Aminoglycosides are active against aerobic gram-negative bacteria. Synergism with β-lactam antibiotics. Adverse effects include ototoxicity, nephrotoxicity, and neuromuscular paralysis.

- Extended interval (i.e., infrequent dosing) regimens are generally recommended. Exceptions include pregnancy, dialysis, CrCl <20, and endocarditis where traditional based dosing is recommended.

Extended Interval Aminoglycoside Nomogram

- Initial dose:
  Gentamicin, 5 mg/kg.
  Tobramycin, 5 mg/kg.
  Amikacin, 15 mg/kg.
- Use IBW to calculate dose. IBW = 50 kg + 2.3 (height [inches] – 60). If >20% above IBW, use formula IBW + 0.4 (actual body weight – IBW).

CRCL (ML/MIN)	INTERVAL
>60	24 hours
40–59	36 hours
20–39	48 hours
<20	Use traditional dosing

- Obtain mid-interval drug level 8–12 hours after the initial dose, then evaluate based on nomogram.
- Repeat drug level 1–2 times weekly and monitor serum creatinine 2–3 times weekly.

FIGURE 15-1. Extended interval aminoglycoside nomogram. (From Barnes-Jewish Hospital Department of Pharmacy. St. Louis: Washington University Medical Center, 1996.)

Traditional Aminoglycoside Dosing

Loading Dose
- Gentamicin, tobramycin
  1.5–2.0 mg/kg dose based on levels
- Amikacin
  5.0–7.5 mg/kg dose based on levels

Maintenance dose is a PERCENTAGE of the selected loading dose. Example: 70 kg pt with CrCl=60ml/min and pneumonia. LD=140mg, MD=120mg q12h.

CrCl (ml/min)	t1/2 (hr)	q8h	q12h	q24h
>90	3.1	84%	100%	-
80	3.4	80%	91%	-
70	3.9	76%	88%	-
60	4.5	-	84%	-
50	5.3	-	79%	-
40	6.5	-	-	92%
30	8.4	-	-	86%
25	9.9	-	-	81%
20	11.9	-	-	75%

For CrCl < 20 ml/min, give loading dose, then follow levels and redose when level drops below 2 mcg/ml.

FIGURE 15-2. Traditional nomogram. (From Barnes-Jewish Hospital Department of Pharmacy. St. Louis: Washington University Medical Center, 1996.)

ANTICOAGULATION

. . . No bleed should be your creed. . . .
Before initiating anticoagulant therapy, ensure that the patient has no history of active peptic ulcers, recent stroke or bleeding, or recent surgery. All patients should have a digital rectal examination and documented guaiac status of examination.

Heparin Weight-Based Nomogram (Unfractionated)

- Initial bolus
  60 U/kg (maximum of 5,000 U)
- Infusion rate
  14 U/kg/hr

A PTT should be ordered 6 hours after initial bolus and 6 hours after each rate change. After two consecutive PTTs are therapeutic (45–70 secs), the PTT should be monitored each morning. In addition, CBC with platelets should be monitored every other day while on IV heparin.

PTT	BOLUS	INFUSION RATE
<40	2,000 U	Increase by 2 U/kg/hr
40–44	None	Increase by 1 U/kg/hr
45–70	None	No change
71–80	None	Decrease by 1 U/kg/hr
81–90	Hold for ½ hour	Decrease by 2 U/kg/hr
>90	Hold for 1 hour	Decrease by 3 U/kg/hr

Guidelines for Antithrombotic Therapy in Heart Valve Replacement

- Tissue or St. Judes in aortic position (2.0–3.0)
  1. Tissue—3 months of coumadin therapy INR
  2. St. Judes in aortic position—lifelong
- Mechanical (except St. Judes in aortic position) INR (2.5–3.5)
  1. Mechanical—lifelong
  2. Consider adding ASA for caged-ball or caged disc valves

Treatment of High INR

INR 5.0–6.9 without Bleeding

- Hold warfarin, search for occult bleed, D/C all other antithrombotic/antiplatelet therapy, and follow INR.

INR 7.0–9.9 without Bleeding
- Hold warfarin; administer vitamin K, 1.0–2.5 mg PO; and document decrease in INR in 48 hours. Give additional vitamin K if INR remains high.

INR >10 without Bleeding
- Hold warfarin; give vitamin K, 3 mg SQ; follow INR every 8 hours; and repeat vitamin K as needed.
- Consider admitting the patient if close follow-up is not possible.

Minor Bleeding
- Hold warfarin; give vitamin K, 1–5 mg SQ; follow INR every 8 hours; and repeat vitamin K as needed.

Major Bleeding
- Hold warfarin; admit patient; give vitamin K, 10 mg SQ, and FFP; follow INR every 6 hours; and repeat vitamin K until INR is normal or bleeding has stopped. Control bleeding as needed through transfusions, surgery, etc.

16

Tools of the Trade
(Fluids, Electrolytes, Vital Signs, Electrocardiography, Radiology)

■ FLUIDS AND BASIC ELECTROLYTES

Basal Requirements

. . . To start 'em up . . .

Water

- Basal water requirement may be calculated as follows:
  For the first 10 kg of body weight, 4 mL/kg/hr plus,
     for the second 10 kg of body weight, 2 mL/kg/hr plus,
     for remaining weight above 20 kg, 1 mL/kg/hr.
- Fever, increased respiratory rate, and sweating can all increase insensible water losses. Insensible losses increase by 100–150 mL/day for each degree of body temperature above 37°C.

Electrolytes

- Sodium: 50–150 mmol/day (as NaCl). Most of this is excreted in the urine.
- Chloride: 50–150 mmol/day (as NaCl).
- Potassium: 20–60 mmol/day (as KCl), assuming renal function is normal. Most of this is excreted in the urine.

Carbohydrates

- Dextrose, 100–150 g/day.
- IV dextrose administration minimizes protein catabolism and prevents ketoacidosis.

Maintenance Intravenous Fluids

. . . To keep 'em going . . .

- Basal requirements of water, electrolytes, and carbohydrates can be conveniently administered as 0.45% NaCl in 5% dextrose plus 20 mmol/L KCl.
- Fluid losses can be divided as urinary losses and all other losses. Urinary losses for the average adult are 0.5–1.0 cc/kg/hr (e.g., 70 kg person produces approximately 40–60 cc/hr or 1200 cc/day). Other losses (water lost in sweat, stool, hydration, insensible losses) total approximately 800 cc/day.
- For average sized adults, 2–3 L (90–125 mL/hr) of this IV solution per day is sufficient (i.e., $D_5 \frac{1}{2}$ NS + 20 mEq KCl @ 100 mL/hr).
- Patients with hypovolemia require more aggressive fluid resuscitation, generally with 0.9% NaCl.

- GI and renal losses may significantly increase the loss of water, Na^+, and K^+. Serum electrolytes should be followed closely in these situations.

■ ELECTROLYTE ABNORMALITIES
. . . If it's high, lower it. If it's low, get it back up. Easy to say, sometimes not so easy to do . . .

Hyponatremia
. . . Please pass the salt . . .

Etiology
- **Hypotonic hyponatremia** is usually caused by primary water gain or Na^+ loss. Na^+ loss may be the result of renal or extrarenal causes.
- **Hypertonic hyponatremia** is caused by an increase in extracellular solute concentration (e.g., hyperglycemia or IV mannitol administration).
- **Isotonic hyponatremia (pseudohyponatremia)** occurs as a result of a decrease in the aqueous phase of plasma (e.g., hyperproteinemia, hyperlipidemia). The concentration of Na^+ per liter of plasma water is normal.

Evaluation
- A careful H&P should be done, paying close attention to fluid status and the neurologic examination.
- Plasma osmolality, urine osmolality, and urine Na^+ should be measured.
- Refer to Fig. 16-1.

Treatment
- Mild asymptomatic hyponatremia generally requires no treatment.
- Careful consideration should be given to the rate of correction of the serum [Na^+]. Too rapid correction may result in osmotic demyelination or central pontine myelinolysis.
- Rapidly developing hyponatremia tends to develop with CNS symptoms and requires more rapid correction. **Severe** symptomatic hyponatremia should be treated with hypertonic saline. The rate of increase of the plasma [Na^+] should not exceed 1–2 mmol/L/hr and no more than 8 mmol/L in the first 24 hours.
- If acute or severe with symptoms, correct [Na^+] to 120–125 in first 24 hours, usually with hypertonic saline, and then gradually until completely corrected over 3–5 days.
- The quantity of [Na^+] required to increase the plasma [Na^+] by a given amount can be estimated as follows:

[Na^+] deficit (mmol) = desired change in [Na^+] × TBW

TBW = 0.6 × body weight (kg).

- For example, if the desired change in [Na^+] is 8 mmol in a 70 kg patient, then 336 mmol of [Na^+] would be required (42 × 8 = 336). This would be 0.65 L hypertonic (3%) saline (336 mmol ÷ 513 mmol/L) or 2.2 L isotonic (0.9%) saline (336 mmol ÷ 154 mmol/L).

FIGURE 16-1. Evaluation of hyponatremia.

Hypernatremia

. . . Hold the salt . . .

Etiology

- Hypernatremia is caused by Na^+ gain or water deficit.
- **Water deficit caused by decreased intake** may be seen in patients with limited access to water (e.g., mental status alteration, intubated patients) or impaired thirst.
- **Water loss may be the result of renal or extrarenal causes.**
- Rarely, hypernatremia may result from **excess Na^+ intake** (e.g., hypertonic saline or $NaHCO_3$).

Evaluation

- A careful H&P should be done, paying close attention to fluid status and the neurologic examination.
- Plasma osmolality, urine osmolality, and urine [Na^+] should be measured.
- Solute excretion rate = urine osmolality × urine volume.
- Refer to Fig. 16-2.

Treatment

- Underlying conditions should be treated (e.g., hyperglycemia, diarrhea, etc.).
- EF volume should be restored in hypovolemic patients with isotonic saline.

$$\text{Body water deficit (L)} = \frac{(\text{plasma } [Na^+] - 140)}{140} \times \text{TBW (L)}$$

$$\text{TBW} = 0.6 \times \text{body weight (kg)}$$

- As with hyponatremia, too rapid correction of hypernatremia is potentially dangerous. The rate of correction of the plasma [Na^+] should not exceed 0.5 mmol/L/hr and the [Na^+] should decrease by no more than 12 mmol/L over the first 24 hours (or no faster than one-half of the volume deficit in the initial 24 hours).
- Don't forget to take into account ongoing losses. The safest route is PO or NG tube administration of water. Alternatively, one-half NS (0.45%), one-quarter NS (0.225%), or DSW can be given IV. Reassess volume status and Na every 8–12 hours.
- Central diabetes insipidus is treated with intranasal DDAVP.
- Nephrogenic diabetes insipidus may be reversible by treating the underlying disorder or eliminating the offending drug (e.g., lithium).

FIGURE 16-2. Evaluation of hypernatremia.

Hypokalemia

. . . More bananas, please . . .

- Defined as a $[K^+]$ <3.5 mmol/L, the clinical features vary greatly. Myalgias and weakness are common complaints. Severe hypokalemia can result in an increased risk of arrhythmias. The $[K^+]$ level of cardiac patients is generally maintained above 4.0.

Etiology

- Hypokalemia may be caused by **decreased intake**. It is infrequently the sole cause, but can exacerbate other causes of hypokalemia.

- **Intracellular shifts** (metabolic alkalosis, insulin, stress-induced catecholamine release, β-adrenergic agonists, anabolic states) may result in hypokalemia.
- K^+ depletion may also be caused by **nonrenal and renal loss**. Renal loss of K^+ may be caused by increased distal K^+ secretion or increased distal tubular flow rate.
- The transtubular potassium gradient may be useful to differentiate types of renal K^+ loss. It is calculated as follows:

$$\text{Transtubular potassium gradient} = \frac{U}{P}K \div \frac{U}{P}osm$$

Calculation assumes $U_{osm} > P_{osm}$.

Evaluation

FIGURE 16-3. Evaluation of hypokalemia. TTKG, transtubular potassium gradient.

Treatment

- K^+ may be repleted either orally or intravenously. It is difficult to provide an algorithmic approach to replacing K^+ as the degree of depletion does not correlate well with plasma levels.
- It is generally safer and more cost effective to replace K^+ via the oral route. Caution should be used in replacing K^+ in patients with renal insufficiency. A reasonable estimate is that every 10 mEq of KCl will increase the serum level 0.05–0.1 mEq/L.
- Severe hypokalemia or patients who cannot take anything PO should be treated with IV KCl. The rate of infusion should not exceed 20 mmol/hr.

Hyperkalemia

. . . So much Kayexalate, so little time . . .
- Defined as a $[K^+]$ in excess of 5.0 mmol/L, the most serious effect is cardiac toxicity. If a suspicious result is received, consider repeating it stat; a potassium can be obtained on an ABG. An ECG must be obtained. Refer to ECG interpretation section later in this chapter. Look for peaked T waves, prolonged PR interval, and QRS duration. Consider continuous cardiac monitoring if the potassium is >6.5.

Etiology

- **Pseudohyperkalemia** is caused by K^+ movement out of cells associated with venipuncture. This may be seen with repeated fist clenching, prolonged tourniquet time, hemolysis, leukocytosis, or thrombocytosis.
- **Increased K^+ intake** is an unusual cause of hyperkalemia, but may be seen with excess K^+ replacement, renal insufficiency, or both.
- **Transcellular shifts** of K^+ may cause hyperkalemia. This may be seen with acidosis, insulin deficiency, drugs (succinylcholine, β-blockers), hypertonicity (e.g., hyperglycemia), hemolysis, tumor lysis, rhabdomyolysis, and hyperkalemic periodic paralysis.
- **Decreased renal K^+ excretion** is the usual cause of chronic hyperkalemia.

Major Causes of Decreased Renal Potassium Excretion

- Renal failure
- Volume depletion
- Primary hypoaldosteronism
- Secondary hypoaldosteronism (e.g., diabetes, mild renal failure, chronic tubulointerstitial disease)
- Drugs (e.g., nonsteroidal antiinflammatory drugs, ACE inhibitor, angiotensin receptor blockers, heparin, spironolactone, triamterene, amiloride, trimethoprim, pentamidine)
- Tubulointerstitial disease (e.g., systemic lupus erythematosus, sickle cell disease, multiple myeloma)
- Type 4 renal tubular acidosis

Evaluation

- Rule out pseudohyperkalemia by repeating the serum electrolytes. Consider drawing the sample without the use of a tourniquet or fist clenching.
- If the patient has thrombocytosis or marked leukocytosis, the sample may be drawn in a heparinized tube.
- Obtain a stat ECG and an ABG (if acidosis is a concern).
- Assess the patient's urine output and renal function.
- Examine the patient, paying particular attention to ECF volume status.
- Review the patient's medication list.
- Determination of plasma renin and aldosterone levels may be useful.

Treatment

- Stop all exogenous K^+ and potentially offending drugs.
- Severe hyperkalemia or hyperkalemia with ECG changes requires emergent treatment. **Do not do this by yourself.** Call your resident immediately.
- **Acute treatment**
  - **Calcium gluconate** 10%, 10 mL IV over 2–3 minutes decreases cardiac membrane excitability. The effect occurs in minutes but lasts only 30–60 minutes. It can be repeated after 5–10 minutes if the ECG does not change. Use with extreme caution in patients receiving digoxin.
  - **Insulin**, 10–20 units IV, causes an intracellular shift of K^+ in 10–30 minutes. The effect lasts for several hours. **Glucose**, 50 gms, should also be administered to prevent hypoglycemia.
  - **$NaHCO_3$**, 1 ampule IV can also be used to cause an intracellular shift of K^+, and the effect can last several hours. This treatment should probably be reserved for patients with severe hyperkalemia and metabolic acidosis. Patients with end-stage renal disease seldom respond and may not tolerate the Na^+ load.
  - **β_2-Adrenergic agonists** are occasionally used to cause an intracellular shift of K^+.
  - **Diuretics** (e.g., furosemide, 40–120 mg IV) enhance K^+ excretion provided renal function is adequate.
  - **Cation exchange resins** (sodium polystyrene sulfonate, Kayexalate) enhance K^+ excretion from the GI tract. Kayexalate may be given PO (20–50 g in 100–200 mL 20% sorbitol) or as a retention enema (50 g in 200 mL 20% sorbitol). The effect may not be evident for several hours and lasts 4–6 hours. Doses may be repeated every 4–6 hours as needed.
  - **Dialysis** may be necessary for severe hyperkalemia when other measures are ineffective and for patients with renal failure.
- **Chronic treatment** is aimed at the underlying condition. Dietary K^+ should be restricted. Metabolic acidosis should be corrected. AntiK^+ drugs should be avoided. Administration of exogenous mineralocorticoid may be effective for select patients.

■ VITAL SIGNS

. . . Occupational hazard: pager-induced intern tachycardia and tachypnea . . .

Although it often seems that the nursing personnel are much more concerned about alterations in vital signs than the physicians, you should take all such calls seriously. If the nurse seems really concerned, you should just go see the patient and assess the situation for yourself.

Blood Pressure

- You will frequently be called with high and low BPs. Be sure you know what the patient's baseline BP has been and recheck the BP yourself before rendering a judgment.
- It is also important to know if the patient is taking any antihypertensive drugs and if they have been given recently.
- **Marked hypotension** should be dealt with emergently. Go see the patient immediately; do not attempt to handle this by phone. Be sure to recheck the BP yourself and assess the other vital signs. The evaluation and management of hypotension is discussed in Chapter 12. Above all, if you find that you're in over your head, call your resident immediately.
- You will often be called regarding **relative hypotension** and whether certain medications should be given (e.g., β-blockers, ACE inhibitors, calcium channel blockers, diuretics). As a general rule, if the patient is asymptomatic and the medications necessary (e.g., for congestive heart failure), the medications may be given. If multiple medications are to be given, consider giving some now and some later.
- Calls for high BP are annoyingly frequent. Resist the temptation to treat **modest elevations**. This is particularly true in patients with a recent stroke.
- Patients with **marked elevations** of BP should be seen immediately. Recheck the BP yourself (be sure the cuff is large enough for the patient's arm) in both arms. Evaluation and management of hypertension are discussed further in Chapter 12.
- If you decide to acutely treat the increased BP, administer oral clonidine, 0.2 mg followed by 0.1 mg PO every hour to a total of 0.7 mg, or until the systolic BP has decreased by 20 mm Hg or more. The BP should be rechecked frequently.
- Alternatively, if the patient is already taking an antihypertensive agent, consider giving an additional dose or the next dose early.

Heart Rate

- An ECG should be done in all with bradycardia or tachycardia. Tachyarrhythmias and bradyarrhythmias are discussed in detail in the ECG Interpretation section, later in this chapter.

- Nursing may wish to hold β-blockers and calcium channel blockers in the setting of relative bradycardia. If the patient is asymptomatic and the heart rate at least 60, they can usually be given. You may consider reducing the dose or giving the medications at different times.

Respiratory Rate

- **Tachypnea** should always be taken seriously; it is a *must see*. It is almost always associated with shortness of breath, which is discussed in Chapter 12.
- A markedly **reduced respiratory rate** is equally serious. Again be sure to measure it yourself (count for a full minute).
- Observe the respiratory pattern closely. Is there a Cheyne-Stokes pattern, which can drastically alter the respiratory rate? Was the patient asleep when the low respiratory rate was recorded? What is the patient's mental status now? Is the patient's airway open and secure? Is the patient taking sedative medications (e.g., narcotics)?
- Checking the O_2 saturation is a good idea, but it tells you nothing about the P_{CO_2}. An ABG is much more informative.

Temperature

- Fever is one of the most common calls an intern receives. Why does it seem this always happens at 4:00 p.m. or 4:00 a.m.? (*But, don't lose your cool. . . .*)
- The evaluation and management of fever are discussed in Chapter 12.

■ ELECTROCARDIOGRAPHIC INTERPRETATION

. . . NSR, no abnormalities—an intern's dream . . .
This section assumes a basic understanding of ECG reading and does not review the fundamentals.

Narrow Complex Tachycardias

Narrow complex tachycardia

Irregular rhythm

- Atrial fibrillation
- Multifocal atrial tachycardia

Regular rhythm

- Sinus tachycardia
- AV node reentrant tachycardia
- Atrial flutter

Sinus Tachycardia
Key Features
- The P wave is of the usual morphology and rates range from 100–160 bpm.
- The QRS maintains its baseline appearance, but rate-related aberrancy occasionally occurs.
- It does not develop or resolve in a paroxysmal fashion.

Management
➤ Treatment is aimed at the underlying cause (e.g., anxiety, pain, hypovolemia, hypoxemia, ischemia, fever, hyperthyroidism, PE).

Atrioventricular Nodal Reentrant Tachycardia
Key Features
- Probably the most common cause of paroxysmal regular SVT.
- Requires two physiologically distinct pathways of conduction (one fast and one slow) in the AV node.
- During NSR, conduction through the AV node occurs over the fast pathway.
- The rate is usually between 150 and 250 bpm.
- The QRS is usually narrow, but can be widened because of a preexisting conduction delay (e.g., BBB) or rate-related aberrancy.
- In **common (typical or slow-fast) AVNRT** there is antegrade conduction over the slow pathway and retrograde conduction back to the atria over the fast pathway, completing the reentrant circuit. Negative P waves are usually simultaneous with the QRS but may rarely be seen in II, III, and aVF. It is usually initiated by an APC.
- In the much more **uncommon (atypical or fast-slow) AVNRT** the circuit is reversed. Negative P waves are usually seen in II, III, and aVF. It is usually initiated by a VPC.

Management
➤ Initial treatment of acute episodes in hemodynamically stable patients begins with vagal maneuvers (e.g., Valsalva's, carotid massage).
➤ If this is unsuccessful, adenosine (6 mg IV followed by 12 mg IV if necessary) should be tried.
➤ Patients who are hemodynamically unstable should be electrically cardioverted.

Preexcitation Syndromes
Key Features
- Requires the presence of an accessory pathway.
- Approximately one-fourth of accessory pathways are concealed and conduct in a retrograde fashion only.
- When the accessory pathway is able to conduct in an antegrade manner during SR, preexcitation (early activation of the ventricles)

occurs. This results in a short PR and a delta wave (initial slurring of the QRS), the Wolff-Parkinson-White syndrome (WPW) (Fig. 16-4).

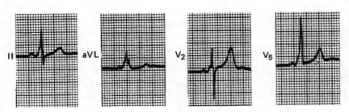

FIGURE 16-4. Wolff-Parkinson-White syndrome with preexcitation.

- During **orthodromic AVRT** conduction is antegrade through the AV node and His-Purkinje system and retrograde through the accessory pathway, completing the reentrant circuit. It may occur with a concealed pathway or in WPW. Rates range from 150–250 bpm. The QRS can maintain its baseline appearance but may also show rate-related aberrancy. Inverted P waves may be seen at the end of the QRS complex. It is paroxysmal, often initiated by an APC or VPC.
- Patients with WPW can also have an **antidromic AVRT** in which conduction in the reentrant circuit is reversed (antegrade through the accessory pathway and retrograde through the AV node and His-Purkinje system). The QRS is also wide in this instance, but this is actually less common than WPW with orthodromic AVRT and aberrant conduction.
- AF and atrial flutter in patients with WPW can be serious because of fast conduction rates and the propensity to initiate VF.

Management

➢ Narrow complex orthodromic AVRT can be treated the same as AVNRT.

➢ Treatment of wide complex tachycardias requires careful consideration. Unless it is orthodromic AVRT with aberrancy (which can be impossible to determine based on a surface ECG), treatment with drugs that slow AV conduction (i.e., adenosine and calcium-channel blockers) may actually increase the ventricular rate with disastrous consequences. When hemodynamically stable, IV procainamide should be used. If you don't know what you're dealing with (and you probably won't), **get help as soon as possible**. If hemodynamically unstable, the patient should be electrically cardioverted.

Atrial Tachycardia

Key Features

- A single different P-wave morphology is seen in **unifocal atrial tachycardia**. Rate is usually between 100 and 200 bpm. The QRS usually maintains its baseline appearance but aberrancy can occur. It is an uncommon cause of SVT.

- In **multifocal atrial tachycardia (MAT)** there are at least three separate P-wave morphologies; the rate is over 100 bpm and irregular. There is variation in the PR interval. It is most often seen in acutely ill elderly patients with pulmonary disease or CHF.

Management

➤ When not associated with digitalis toxicity, unifocal atrial tachycardia may be treated with calcium channel blockers or β-blockers.

➤ Treatment of MAT is focused on the underlying condition.

Atrial Fibrillation

Key Features

- Atrial activity is completely disorganized. The baseline is wavy without clear P waves (Fig. 16-5).
- The ventricular rate is irregularly irregular and may be slow to fast (usually >100 bpm in untreated patients).
- The QRS typically maintains its usual morphology. Variable rate-related aberrancy may also be seen.
- The incidence of AF increases with age and there are many possible causes including CAD, MI, valvular disease, PE, COPD, pericarditis, hyperthyroidism or hypothyroidism, acute alcohol intoxication, and idiopathic.

FIGURE 16-5. Atrial fibrillation.

Management

➤ If the patient is unstable (infarction, ischemia, hypotension, PE, mental status alteration) immediate electrical cardioversion is indicated.

➤ When the patient is stable, rate control may be achieved with AV nodal blocking agents.

➤ Diltiazem, 0.25 mg/kg IVP over 2 minutes; if no response repeat 0.35 mg/kg IVP over 2 minutes; follow with an IV infusion at 5–15 mg/hr. Diltiazem is probably the agent of choice in most patients.

➤ Metoprolol, 5 mg IVP every 5 minutes to a total of 15 mg followed by oral dosing.

➤ Verapamil, 5–10 mg IVP over 2 minutes, may repeat after 15–30 minutes. Verapamil is more likely to cause hypotension and congestive heart failure. When given IV, it can only be given in bolus doses.

➢ Digoxin, 0.25–0.50 mg IVP; then 0.125–0.25 mg IVP every 4–6 hours to a total dose of 0.75–1.35 mg; followed by oral dosing. Digoxin's effect will take longer than other agents. It can be a good choice in patients with a reduced ejection fraction.

➢ Pharmacotherapy for AF with WPW and preexcitation is of special concern (see previous discussion).

➢ In stable patients, anticoagulation is generally recommended before cardioversion (chemical or electrical) if AF has been present for >48 hours or the duration is unknown.

Atrial Flutter

Key Features

- Atrial flutter is characterized by flutter waves in a regular, undulating, sawtooth pattern at a rate of 280–350 bpm. Flutter waves are best seen in leads II, III, aVF, and V_1 (Fig. 16-6).
- The ventricular rate depends on the degree of AV block (2:1, 3:1) and may be regular or variable.
- Vagal maneuvers may slow AV conduction, revealing the flutter waves.
- The QRS maintains its baseline appearance.
- Atrial flutter is most commonly seen in those conditions associated with AF (see previous discussion).

FIGURE 16-6. Atrial flutter.

Management

➢ Management of atrial flutter is similar to that for AF.

➢ Patients who are unstable should be immediately electrically cardioverted.

➢ Rate control in stable patients may be achieved in a similar manner as for AF.

Wide Complex Tachycardias

Wide complex tachycardias may be of either supraventricular or ventricular origin. Differentiation of SVT with aberrant conduction from VT on the basis of the surface ECG may be difficult (if not impossible in some patients). This differentiation is not merely academic but critical to appropriate treatment. If you find yourself in this predicament, **call for help immediately**. Regardless of the cause, if the patient is unstable (ischemia or infarction, hypotension, CHF, altered mental status), electrical cardioversion is indicated.

Ventricular Tachycardia

. . . This is bad. Really bad. Call for backup now. . . .

Key Features

- VT is the most frequent life-threatening arrhythmia, and it is most often associated with MI.
- VT is defined as ≥ three ventricular complexes in a row at a rate of 100–250. Sustained VT lasts longer than 30 seconds or is associated with hemodynamic collapse.
- The QRS is ≥120 milliseconds and often has an LBBB pattern. The T wave is usually in the opposite direction of the main QRS deflection (Fig. 16-7). It may be monomorphic (single QRS morphology) or polymorphic (multiple QRS morphologies).
- AV dissociation is present but usually cannot be easily seen.
- There may be occasional capture, fusion beats, or both.
- VT is often associated with hemodynamic compromise and has a distressing tendency to degenerate into VF and death.
- VT can easily be confused with SVT with rate-related aberrancy or a preexistent intraventricular conduction defect, antidromic AVRT, and preexcited AF (see previous discussion).

FIGURE 16-7. Ventricular tachycardia.

Management

➤ If a wide complex tachycardia cannot be immediately and definitively diagnosed, it should initially be treated as VT, and you should call for help at once!

➤ Sustained VT (or any other wide complex tachycardia) in unstable patients requires immediate DC cardioversion by ACLS protocol.

➤ Pharmacologic treatment may be attempted in stable VT patients using procainamide, lidocaine, bretylium, or amiodarone. Of course, you'll call for help before you do this!

Torsades de Pointes

Key Features

- TDP is a rapid, polymorphic VT with QRS complexes that oscillate in amplitude and morphology, producing the appearance of a continuously twisting axis of depolarization.

- It is usually preceded by an prolonged QT interval and initiated by a PVC.
- It may be associated with electrolyte-induced long QT (most notably hypokalemia and hypomagnesemia), drugs that prolong the QT, congenital long QT syndromes, and end-stage cardiomyopathy.
- It often occurs for brief periods but can be sustained with hemodynamic collapse.

Management

➤ Sustained, unstable TDP should be treated with electrical cardioversion.

➤ Offending drugs should be stopped and electrolyte abnormalities should be corrected.

➤ IV MgSO$_4$ 1–2 g (up to 4–6 g) can be highly effective, even if the magnesium level is normal.

Ventricular Fibrillation

. . . Close this book immediately! There should be multiple people running toward the patient with powerful electrical equipment. . . .

Key Features

- VF is characterized by completely chaotic, rapid, highly variable amplitude electrical activity emanating from the ventricles. There are no discernible QRS complexes.
- There is no effective cardiac output and if untreated, rapidly results in death.

Management

➤ All patients require immediate electrical cardioversion by ACLS protocol.

Conduction Abnormalities

First-Degree Atrioventricular Block

Key Features

- The PR interval is lengthened (>200 milliseconds), but all P waves are conducted to the ventricles (Fig. 16-8).
- It is associated with increased vagal tone, conduction system degeneration, ischemia, drugs (e.g., antiarrhythmics, calcium channel blockers, β-blockers), and electrolyte abnormalities.

FIGURE 16-8. First-degree AV block.

Management

➤ Primary AV block is almost always asymptomatic and rarely requires any specific treatment.

Second-Degree Atrioventricular Block, Mobitz Type I (Wenckebach's Disease)

Key Features

- Not all of the atrial impulses are conducted.
- There is a progressive delay in AV conduction before a completely blocked P wave. This results in a progressive prolongation of the PR interval and shortening of the RR interval before a nonconducted P wave (Fig. 16-9).
- The QRS complexes maintain their baseline appearance and appear in regular groupings. This grouping should immediately raise suspicion for Mobitz type I second-degree AV block.
- The site of conduction block is almost always within the AV node.
- Etiologies are the same as for primary AV block including ischemia (particularly in the inferior or posterior distribution).
- It is usually benign and generally does not degenerate to complete heart block.

FIGURE 16-9. Mobitz type I (Wenckebach), second-degree AV block.

Management

➤ Mobitz type I second-degree AV block is usually asymptomatic and transient. Treatment is generally not necessary.

➤ If symptomatic, atropine (0.5–1.0 mg IV repeated every 3–5 minutes prn to a total dose of 0.04 mg/kg) may be given and if persistent, cardiac pacing may be necessary.

Second-Degree Atrioventricular Block, Mobitz Type II

Key Features

- Not all of the atrial impulses are conducted; however, there is no preceding conduction block.
- The PR interval is fixed and usually normal, with suddenly and intermittently blocked P waves (Fig. 16-10).
- Blocked conduction may occur at a fixed ratio (e.g., 2:1, 3:1, 4:1).

- The site of conduction block is usually infranodal within the His-Purkinje system.
- Causes include increased vagal tone, conduction system disease, antiarrhythmic drugs, and ischemia (particularly in the anterior distribution).
- Mobitz type II second-degree AV block usually implies severe conduction system disease and often precedes the development of complete heart block, especially when a bundle branch block is also present. Therefore, you should always take this conduction service very seriously.

FIGURE 16-10. Mobitz type II, second-degree AV block.

Management

➤ Symptomatic patients should initially be treated with atropine (0.5–1.0 mg IV repeated every 3–5 minutes prn to a total dose of 0.04 mg/kg), but the response is typically poor and temporary.
➤ Pacemaker placement is frequently indicated, regardless of whether the patient is symptomatic.

Third-Degree (Complete) Atrioventricular Block

Key Features

- As the name implies, AV block is complete and no P waves are conducted to the ventricles (Fig. 16-11).
- An automatic focus below the block takes over at its own intrinsic rate (usually slower than the P wave rate, <50).
- There is no fixed relationship between the P waves and the QRS complexes (AV dissociation).
- The QRS complexes are usually wide, but may be narrow if they arise from a junctional focus.
- The site of conduction block may be AV node or more typically within the His-Purkinje system.
- Third-degree AV block may be congenital or acquired. Etiologies of acquired complete heart block include idiopathic conduction system degeneration, ischemia or infarct, infiltrative diseases, drug toxicity, calcific aortic stenosis, endocarditis, and cardiac surgery.

Management

➤ Emergent treatment with atropine (0.5–1.0 mg IV repeated every 3–5 minutes prn to a total dose of 0.04 mg/kg), and pacemaker placement is usually required.

FIGURE 16-11. Complete heart block.

Myocardial Ischemia and Infarction

Key Features

- Myocardial ischemia is characterized by symmetric T-wave inversion that may be slight to deep, flat or down-sloping ST depression, or both.
- The ECG typically demonstrates sequential changes during the evolution of an acute Q-wave MI. Certainly not all patients show this typical sequence, and the time course of the changes may vary among patients.
- In the earliest hyperacute phase tall and prolonged T waves are seen.
- This is followed by the acute phase of convex-up ST-segment elevation in the leads facing the area of injury.
- Reciprocal ST depression may be seen in the leads opposite to the area of infarction.
- Over the following hours to days, the R-wave amplitude decreases and pathologic Q waves appear (>40 milliseconds or greater than or equal to one-third of the entire QRS amplitude).
- As the ST segments return to baseline, the T waves become symmetrically inverted.
- Over time, the T waves may return to their baseline orientation.
- The distribution of these typical ECG changes can be used to predict the location of the myocardial infarction (Table 16-1). It is important to remember, however, that this method of localization can be rather imprecise (Fig. 16-12).
- The ST segments may remain chronically elevated in the setting of LV aneurysm formation.
- Noninfarction-related Q waves can be seen in myocarditis, cardiomyopathies, muscular dystrophies, scleroderma, amyloidosis, sarcoidosis, WPW, LVH, BBB, COPD, and PE.
- Non-ST elevation MIs often have much more nonspecific and subtle ECG changes. Possible changes include persistent ST depression, ST elevation without development of Q waves, T-wave inversions, loss of QRS amplitude, and poor R-wave progression across the precordium.

TABLE 16-1. ELECTROCARDIOGRAPHIC LOCALIZATION OF MYOCARDIAL INFARCTION

Area of MI	ECG Abnormality	Artery Involved
Septal	ST elevation and Q waves V_1–V_2	Proximal left anterior descending, septal perforators
Anteroseptal	ST elevation and Q waves V_1–V_4	Left anterior descending
Anterior	ST elevation and Q waves V_3–V_4	Left anterior descending
Anterolateral	ST elevation and Q waves I, aVL, V_3–V_6	Mid-left anterior descending or circumflex
Extensive anterior	ST elevation and Q waves I, aVL, V_1–V_6	Proximal left anterior descending
Lateral	ST elevation and Q waves I, aVL, V_6	Circumflex
High lateral	ST elevation and Q waves I, aVL	Circumflex
Inferior	ST elevation and Q waves II, III, aVF	Right coronary artery
Posterior	Tall R and ST depression V_1–V_2	Right coronary artery or circumflex
Right ventricular	ST elevation V_4R	Proximal right coronary artery

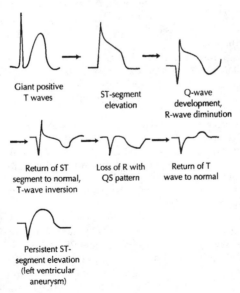

Giant positive T waves → ST-segment elevation → Q-wave development, R-wave diminution

Return of ST segment to normal, T-wave inversion → Loss of R with QS pattern → Return of T wave to normal

Persistent ST-segment elevation (left ventricular aneurysm)

FIGURE 16-12. ST and T-wave changes in MI. (From Alpert J. *Cardiology for the primary care physician.* Appleton and Lange, 1998:168, with permission.)

- Prior MIs and preexistent or newly developed conduction abnormalities may mask or make these typical changes difficult to interpret.
- Other conditions may mimic the ECG changes of an acute MI including pericarditis, myocarditis, and aortic dissection.
- It is very difficult to diagnose acute MI changes in the setting of LBBB or a paced rhythm.

Management

➤ A detailed discussion of the management of myocardial ischemia and infarction is beyond the scope of this manual. Refer to the Chapter 12 section on chest pain and call your resident immediately.

Miscellaneous Conditions

Pericarditis
Key Features

- The acute phase of pericarditis is characterized by diffuse flat or concave-up ST-segment elevation, particularly in the precordial leads. The entire T wave may be lifted off the baseline and there may also be diffuse PR depression (Fig. 16-13).
- In the intermediate phase diffuse T-wave inversion appears and ST elevation resolves.
- In the late phase T-wave inversion resolves.
- There is no development of Q waves.
- Pericarditis has many possible causes including infectious (viral, bacterial, fungal, tuberculous), post-MI, posttraumatic, postpericardiotomy, collagen vascular diseases, drug-induced (hydralazine, procainamide), uremia, infiltrative (sarcoidosis, amyloidosis), neoplastic, radiation, and idiopathic.

FIGURE 16-13. Pericarditis.

Management

➤ Specifically, treatable causes should be managed in the appropriate manner (e.g., antimicrobial agents for infectious causes or dialysis for uremia).
➤ Antiinflammatory treatment may be effective (NSAIDs or prednisone).

➤ Narcotic analgesics may be given for refractory pain.
➤ Patients should be observed closely for the development of cardiac tamponade.
➤ Anticoagulants should be avoided because of the risk of hemopericardium.

Hyperkalemia

Key Features

- The earliest ECG feature of hyperkalemia is tall, peaked, symmetric, narrow-based T waves. These are often referred to as "tented" T waves. They are best seen in leads II, III, and $V_2–V_4$ (Fig. 16-14).
- The P-wave amplitude then decreases and the PR interval becomes prolonged. With increasingly severe hyperkalemia the P waves eventually all but disappear. Consequently, arrhythmias that are common in hyperkalemia can be difficult to identify.
- With severe hyperkalemia the QRS progressively widens, the R amplitude decreases, and S waves become prominent. There may also be ST-segment depression or elevation.
- Eventually, with extreme hyperkalemia the ECG takes on a slow sinusoidal pattern that may degenerate into asystole or VF if not immediately and aggressively treated.

FIGURE 16-14. Hyperkalemia.

Management

➤ The acute management of hyperkalemia is covered in the section regarding electrolyte abnormalities, earlier in this chapter.

Digitalis Effect and Toxicity

Key Features

- At therapeutic levels digitalis may cause a characteristic, gradual down-sloping, concave-up (also described as "scooping" or "sagging") of the ST segment. The ST is typically depressed and shortened and the T wave amplitude decreased. Collectively, this is known as the "dig effect" (Fig. 16-15).
- At times it can be difficult to differentiate the dig effect from other causes of ST depression.
- Digitalis toxicity has been associated with nearly all known arrhythmias. Common digitalis toxicity associated arrhythmias include

sinus block, APCs, PAT with block, JPCs, junctional tachycardia, AV block, VPCs, VT (including bidirectional VT), and VF.
- Hypokalemia, hypomagnesemia, and hypercalcemia may enhance the toxic effects of digitalis.
- Because of its narrow therapeutic window, toxicity can occur even when the digitalis level is within the usual therapeutic range.

FIGURE 16-15. Digitalis effect.

Management

➤ Digitalis should be discontinued immediately.
➤ In the setting of recent acute ingestion of potentially toxic amounts of digitalis and before toxic cardiac side effects have occurred, induced emesis or gastric lavage may be used. Activated charcoal may also be administered to reduce further absorption.
➤ The ECG should be continuously monitored.
➤ Electrolyte abnormalities (particularly hypokalemia) should be carefully corrected. However, care should be taken as rapid increases in potassium (even within the normal range) may worsen AV conduction and lead to complete heart block. Serum potassium concentration should be determined before potassium administration. Massive digitalis overdoses can cause hyperkalemia.
➤ Ventricular arrhythmias can be treated with IV lidocaine (1.0–1.5 mg/kg initial IV bolus, additional 0.5–1.5 mg/kg IV bolus injections prn up to a total of 3 mg/kg, followed by continuous IV infusion at 2–4 mg/minute) or phenytoin (250 mg IV loading dose over 10 minutes, followed by additional 100 mg IV doses every 5 minutes prn to a total of 1,000 mg).
➤ Bradyarrhythmias may be treated with atropine (0.5–1.0 mg IV repeated every 3–5 minutes prn to a total dose of 0.04 mg/kg) or temporary pacing.
➤ Digitalis-specific Fab antibody fragments (Digibind) may be given when other methods have been ineffective. One vial of Fab fragments is equivalent to 40 mg and neutralizes approximately 0.6 mg of digitalis. The dosage is calculated as follows: Number of vials = [dig level (ng/mL) × weight (kg)]/100. The Fab fragments are given in NS over 15–30 minutes.
➤ Electrical cardioversion should be used only as a last resort, when all other measures have failed. Cardioversion in the setting of digitalis toxicity can cause VT or VF that is resistant to any further cardioversion.

■ ACID–BASE DISORDERS

. . . Retention, compensation, deficits . . .

- Changes in acid–base balance occur as a result of changes in [H⁺] and [HCO₃⁻].
- **Acidemia** results from either decreased [HCO₃⁻] or increased P_{CO_2}.
- **Alkalemia** results from either increased [HCO₃⁻] or decreased P_{CO_2}.
- Stepwise approach to an ABG:
  1. Examine the pH. Is the patient acidemic or alkalemic?
  2. Examine the [HCO₃⁻]. In primary metabolic disorders, it moves in the same direction as the pH.
  3. Examine the P_{CO_2}. In primary respiratory disorders, it moves in the opposite direction as the pH.
  4. Is there adequate respiratory or metabolic compensation? (Table 16-2.)
  5. If a metabolic acidosis is present, calculate the anion gap. If no gap is present, calculate the urine anion gap.

TABLE 16-2. PRIMARY ACID–BASE DISORDERS

Disorder	Abnormality	Primary Changes	Compensatory Response
Metabolic acidosis	[HCO₃⁻] loss or [H⁺] gain	↓[HCO₃⁻]	↓P_{CO_2} by 1.0–1.3 mm Hg for every 1.0 mmol/L ↓[HCO₃⁻]
Metabolic alkalosis	[H⁺] loss or [HCO₃⁻] gain	↑[HCO₃⁻]	↑P_{CO_2} 0.6–0.7 mm Hg for every 1 mmol/L ↑[HCO₃⁻]
Respiratory acidosis	Alveolar hypoventilation	↑P_{CO_2}	
Acute			↑[HCO₃⁻] 1.0 mmol/L for every 10 mm Hg ↑P_{CO_2}
Chronic			↑[HCO₃⁻] 3.0–3.5 mmol/L for every 10 mm Hg ↑P_{CO_2}
Respiratory alkalosis	Alveolar hyper-ventilation	↓P_{CO_2}	
Acute			↓[HCO₃⁻] 2.0 mmol/L for every 10 mm Hg ↓P_{CO_2}
Chronic			↓[HCO₃⁻] 4.0–5.0 mmol/L for every 10 mm Hg ↓P_{CO_2}

See the diagram on the inside front cover of this book.

Metabolic Acidosis
TABLE 16-3. CAUSES OF METABOLIC ACIDOSIS

Increased Anion Gap	Normal Anion Gap
Uremia	GI [HCO_3^-] loss (diarrhea, urinary diversion, small bowel, biliary, pancreatic, cholestyramine, or ingestion of Ca or Mg chloride)
Diabetic ketoacidosis; alcoholic ketoacidosis	
Lactic acidosis	Ingestion of exogenous acids
Methanol	Proximal (type 2) renal tubular acidosis
Paraldehyde	Classic distal (type 1) renal tubular acidosis
Ethylene glycol	Hyperkalemic (type 4) renal tubular acidosis
Salicylates	Early renal insufficiency
	Expansion acidosis (rapid saline administration)
	Drug-induced hyperkalemia (K^+-sparing diuretics, trimethoprim, pentamidine, ACE inhibitors, nonsteroidal antiinflammatory drugs, cyclosporine), carbonic anhydrase inhibitors

Treatment
➤ Treatment of the underlying condition should be the primary focus.
➤ Severe acidosis (pH <7.20) may require treatment with parenteral $NaHCO_3$.
➤ The bicarbonate deficit may be calculated as follows:

$$[HCO_3^-] \text{ deficit (mEq/L)} = [0.5 \times \text{body wt (kg)}] - (24 - \text{measured } [HCO_3^-])$$

➤ Rapid infusion should be considered for only severe acidosis.
➤ Overaggressive correction should be avoided to prevent overshoot alkalosis.
➤ Hypernatremia and fluid overload can occur with $NaHCO_3$ administration.
➤ Serum electrolytes should be followed closely.

Metabolic Alkalosis

Etiology
• Metabolic alkalosis may be caused by HCO_3^- gain/H^+ loss or volume contraction.
• Vomiting and diuretic use are the two most common causes (Table 16-4).

TABLE 16-4. CAUSES OF METABOLIC ALKALOSIS

Cl⁻ Responsive (Urine Cl⁻ <10 mmol/L)	Cl⁻ Unresponsive (Urine Cl⁻ >10 mmol/L)
Gastrointestinal	Normotensive
Vomiting, NG suction	K^+ or Mg^{2+} depletion
Villous adenoma	Bartter's syndrome
Congenital chloridorrhea	Hypercalcemia/hypoparathyroidism
Cystic fibrosis	Hypertensive
Renal	Primary aldosteronism
Diuretics	Hyperreninemic hyperaldosteronism
Posthypercapnic state	Adrenal enzyme defects
Nonreabsorbable anions (penicillin)	Cushing's syndrome
Exogenous alkali ($NaHCO_3^-$ massive transfusion, antacids, acetate, citrate)	Exogenous mineralocorticoid
Contraction alkalosis	Pseudohyperaldosteronism (licorice, carbenoxolone, tobacco chewing, Liddle's syndrome)

Treatment

➤ Treatment of the underlying condition should be the primary focus.
➤ When EF volume contraction is present it should be corrected with isotonic NS.
➤ Hypokalemia and hypomagnesemia should be corrected.
➤ Cl⁻ unresponsive causes do not improve with administration of NaCl; in fact, it may be hazardous.
➤ K⁺-sparing diuretics may be effective for some forms of hyperaldosteronism.

Respiratory Acidosis

Etiology

- ↑Pco_2 is almost always the result of alveolar hypoventilation.
- In **acute respiratory acidosis** the pH ↓0.08 for every 10 mm Hg ↑Pco_2 above 40.
- In **chronic respiratory acidosis** the pH ↓0.03 for every 10 mm Hg ↑Pco_2 above 40.
- Renal compensation takes several days to develop fully.

TABLE 16-5. CAUSES OF RESPIRATORY ACIDOSIS

Central respiratory depression (drugs, sleep apnea, obesity, CNS disease)

Airway obstruction (foreign body, laryngospasm, severe bronchospasm)

Neuromuscular abnormalities (polio, kyphoscoliosis, myasthenia, muscular dystrophy)

Parenchymal lung disease (COPD, pneumothorax, pneumonia, pulmonary edema, interstitial lung disease)

Treatment

➤ Treatment is directed at the underlying condition.
➤ Potentially contributing drugs should be stopped or counteracted (e.g., naloxone, flumazenil).
➤ Ventilatory assistance may be required (CPAP or mechanical ventilation).
➤ Generally, $NaHCO_3$ treatment is not given, unless the patient is ventilated and the pH remains severely low.

Respiratory Alkalosis

Etiology

• It is important to remember that tachypnea/hyperventilation does not necessarily imply a simple respiratory alkalosis. If you have any uncertainty, obtain an ABG.

TABLE 16-6. CAUSES OF RESPIRATORY ALKALOSIS

Central stimulation (anxiety, pain, hyperventilation syndrome, head trauma, CVA, tumors, fever/infection, salicylates, thyroxine, progesterone)

Hypoxemia (any causes)

Airway irritation

Decreased lung compliance (CHF, fibrosis)

Pulmonary embolism

Hepatic insufficiency/failure

Pregnancy

Hyperthyroidism

Overzealous mechanical ventilation

Treatment

➤ Treatment is directed at the underlying condition.
➤ Psychogenic hyperventilation may be treated by rebreathing from a paper bag.

■ RADIOGRAPH INTERPRETATION

. . . Know your patients inside out. . . .

Chest X-Ray

The chest x-ray is by far the most common radiograph you will order and need to interpret. When reading a chest x-ray, the most important thing is to be systematic. Be sure to check the name and date on the film and compare with old films whenever possible.

Technique

- Is the exposure correct? Underexposure can cause you to see things that aren't there, while overexposure can cause pathology to disappear. You should be able to faintly see the intervertebral spaces through the cardiac silhouette.
- Is the patient properly positioned? The spinous processes and trachea should be midline. The clavicular heads should be equidistant from the spinous processes. Rotated films distort the appearance of the cardiac silhouette and hila.
- Is the frontal film a PA or AP? AP films are often done in emergent situations or when the patient cannot stand. They can easily cause you to see things that aren't there.
- Was the film taken at full inspiration? If not, you may be seeing things again.

Soft Tissues

- Examine the soft tissues for symmetry, subcutaneous air, edema, and breast tissue.

Bones

- Systematically look at the sternum, ribs, clavicles, spine, and shoulders.
- Look for fractures, osteolytic or osteoblastic lesions, and arthritic changes.

Diaphragm

- The sides of the diaphragm should be equal and slightly rounded. The right side may be slightly higher.
- Look for blunting of the costophrenic angles that suggest small pleural effusions.
- Flat diaphragms suggest emphysema.
- A unilateral high diaphragm may suggest paralysis, loss of lung volume on that side, or eventration.
- Check for free air under the diaphragm.

Heart and Mediastinum

- A maximal heart width greater than half of the chest width suggests cardiomegaly or pericardial effusion.
- The aortic knob should be distinct.

- Mediastinal widening is indicative of thoracic aortic dissection or aneurysm, pericardial effusion, or mass.
- The trachea should be midline and not deviated.
- Mediastinal and tracheal deviation may be seen with pneumothorax.
- Use lateral films to confirm findings on PA and look for retrocardiac infiltrates.

Hilar Structures

- The left hilum is usually 2–3 cm higher than the right. They are generally of equal size.
- Enlarged hila suggest lymphadenopathy.

Lung Fields

- Look for normal lung markings all the way out to the chest wall to rule out pneumothorax. Be sure not to miss this! If you think you've detected a pneumothorax, let your resident know right away.
- Normal lung markings taper as they travel out to the periphery and are smaller in the upper lungs. Lung markings in the upper lung fields that are as large or larger ("cephalization") suggest pulmonary edema.
- Kerley's B lines (small linear densities at the lateral lung bases) are also seen with CHF.
- Hyperlucency of the lung fields is seen in COPD.
- Examine the lung fields for the presence of infiltrates and masses.
- Obliteration of part or all of the heart border (silhouette sign) implies that the lesion is anterior. It may be located in the RML, lingula, or anterior segment of the upper lobe.
- A small pleural effusion is suggested by blunting of the costophrenic angle. Larger effusions obscure the shadow of the diaphragm and produce an upward-curving shadow along the chest wall. A straight horizontal fluid level indicates a concurrent pneumothorax.
- Lateral decubitus films should be done to ensure that the effusion is free flowing and large enough to attempt thoracentesis.

Plain Abdominal Films

Generally speaking, plain abdominal films ("KUB" or "obstructive series") are of limited value. Despite that, they are ordered quite frequently. Again, a systematic approach is key.

Bones

- Examine the bones first or else you'll forget.
- Begin with the spine, then ribs, pelvis, and upper femurs. Look for signs of arthritis, fractures, and osteolytic or osteoblastic lesions.

Soft Tissues

- Systematically study the soft tissues looking for evidence of masses or calcifications.
- Be sure to carefully look for free air under the diaphragm (upright film) or next to the abdominal wall (lateral decubitus film). Free air is indicative of perforation. If you see this, let your resident know immediately!

Gastrointestinal Structures

- Look for the gastric bubble. A large air-distended stomach suggests some form of obstruction.
- Observe the bowel gas pattern. A small amount of air is generally seen in the colon, while the small bowel is generally devoid of air. Fecal material is often visible in the colon although large amounts may be seen in constipation.
- The colon may become greatly distended with air in colonic obstruction (colonic distention proximal to the obstruction) or ileus. Unless the distention is severe, the haustral markings are maintained. (The large bowel markings are differentiated from small bowel markings by their wider spacing, and the incomplete crossing of the lumen). When the ileocecal valve is incompetent, large bowel obstruction may also cause distention of the small bowel.
- Distention of the small bowel may be seen in mechanical obstruction and ileus. Small bowel striations are much more numerous and completely cross the lumen. With mechanical obstruction there is distention proximal to the obstruction and clearing of air distally.
- The appearance of ileus is much less distinct. There is discontinuous air in the small and usually large bowel. The degree of distention is also less remarkable and discontinuous.
- Air–fluid levels do not distinguish mechanical obstruction from ileus. They may be seen in both conditions.

■ PREPARATION FOR PROCEDURES

. . . A procedure canceled due to inadequate prep is like having a hemolyzed specimen. Nobody's happy, you have to do it again, and it's always the intern's fault. . . .

General Points

- Perform plain x-ray films prior to contrast studies. Perform contrast studies prior to barium studies (i.e., start with studies that require greatest amount of clarity of the area in question).
- Consult your radiology department if you have questions about what study to order or to confirm preparation for procedures. Some preparations are institution specific.
- Studies requiring no preparation include: chest x-rays, abdominal x-rays, C-spine series, skull series, transthoracic echo, as well as these listed below.
- Remember to restart the diet post procedure or if procedure is canceled.

Contrast Reactions

- Everyone feels a sense of warmth or flushing during contrast administration—this is not an allergy.
- For known contrast sensitivity (e.g., hives, rash), consider prednisone, 60 mg PO q6 × 4, prior to the exam. Benadryl, 50 mg PO, can also be added.

- Alternatively, consider using prednisone, 60 mg, 12 hrs prior to procedure, then take diphenhydramine, 50 mg + Cimetidine, 300 mg + prednisone, 60 mg, when on call to the procedure.
- Although only non-ionic contrast is used for CT (check your institution for confirmation), if your patient has had a major event with previous contrast administration (e.g., shock or airway compromise), discuss this with the radiologist **prior** to ordering a test.
- The contrast used in MR examinations is a gadolinium preparation, not iodinated contrast. It would be highly unusual for a patient to have an allergy to gadolinium.
- IV hydration and Mucomyst (600 mg bid prior to procedure) may also be added in patients where renal insufficiency is a concern.
- Contrast should not be given to anyone with a Cr >2.0.

Gastrointestinal Radiology

- GI studies can be uncomfortable and do require patient cooperation. If your patient is paralyzed, demented, angry, or has altered mental status, the study will likely be suboptimal.
- General rules for the "barium versus hypaque" dilemma (call the radiologist if you have specific questions):
  1. **Barium** is bad in pleural or peritoneal spaces so avoid this if perforation, obstruction, aspiration, or a fistula is suspected. Do not use if the patient is likely to need a laparotomy soon.
  2. **Hypaque** is bad to aspirate, so avoid in cases of possible aspiration.

PROCEDURE	PREPARATION
CT	
Chest/extremity/head	Usually none, but may need contrast
Abdominal/pelvic	Full liquid diet starting 4 hours prior to procedure
	Oral contrast administration
MRI	None
Ultrasound	
Abdominal	NPO starting 6 hours prior to procedure
Pelvic	4 glasses of water 1 hour prior; no voiding 1 hour prior
Gastrointestinal studies	
Barium swallow (used to evaluate pharynx and esophagus typically for dysphagia work-up)	NPO 1 hour prior to procedure

(continued)

PROCEDURE	PREPARATION
Modified barium swallow (used to evaluate for possible aspiration during feeding)	NPO 1 hour prior to procedure
Upper GI (used to evaluate the esophagus, stomach, and proximal small intestine; typically used to look for ulcers)	NPO starting midnight the day prior to procedure
Small bowel follow-through (contrast is followed through the small intestine; typically used to evaluate for areas of stricture or large mucosal abnormalities)	1 glass of water every hour between 12 and 7 p.m.; no smoking/chewing tobacco after midnight
Barium enema (used to evaluate the colon for mucosal lesions such as polyps and strictures)	Clear liquids 1 day prior; NPO after midnight 1 glass of water every hour from 1 to 7 p.m. 1 day prior, mag citrate at 8 p.m., 4 Dulcolax tablets at 11 p.m., 1 Dulcolax suppository at 7 a.m.
HIDA scan	NPO starting midnight the day prior to procedure
Genitourinary studies	
Cystogram	No dietary restriction Full bladder
Interventional studies	
Venogram	Clear liquids; NPO 1 hour prior to procedure
Lymphangiogram	Light meal prior; limit fluids 2–3 hours prior to procedure
Endoscopic studies	
EGD/ERCP	NPO starting 6 hours prior to procedure
Colonoscopy	Clear liquids 1 day prior to procedure; NPO after midnight, 1 gallon of Go-LYTELY (1 cup per 15 minutes until done; consider NG tube if not able to complete)
Flexible sigmoidoscopy	Clear liquids starting with dinner the night before; NPO after midnight Mag Citrate at 8 p.m., 1 glass of water every 2 hours until 10 p.m., then 3 Dulcolax tablets at 10 p.m., and 1 Dulcolax suppository at 6 a.m.

Cardiac Studies

In general:
- No smoking 2 hours prior to test, remove nicotine patches the morning of the test.
- Small sips of water with medication are fine.

TEST	PREPARATION
Coronary angiogram	NPO after midnight
Stress echo, dobutamine stress echo, or exercise stress test	Take all medications (unless they need to be taken with food)
Nuclear stress test (walking)	Hold a.m. doses of calcium channel blockers and β-blockers
Adenosine nuclear stress test (non-walking)	For diabetics on insulin only, half the normal insulin dose and eat a light meal 3 hours prior to procedure (no fats or dairy products)
	Avoid any xanthine containing products (e.g., chocolate, caffeine) and theophylline or persantine for 24 hours prior to procedure

MRI

- Absolute contraindications are pacemakers and ferromagnetic intracranial aneurysm clips.
- Relative contraindications are recent operations (less than a few weeks) and recent vascular stenting. Prosthetic hip joints or metal implants aren't generally contraindicated, but their artifact may obscure any adjacent lesions.
- As with CT, the patient must be able to lie still and cooperate—consider mild sedation (e.g., Ativan) if necessary. Patients may get claustrophobic.

Ultrasound

- Abdominal ultrasounds can be used to evaluate the gallbladder, liver, and kidneys. The pancreas is typically not well visualized—use CT instead.
- Ultrasound can also locate pockets of fluid to guide paracentesis.
- It is important the patient be made NPO as gas can obstruct the image.

17

Approach to Consultation

. . . With a little help from our friends . . .

■ THE MEDICINE CONSULT

Guiding principles for effective medicine consults were first suggested by Lee Goldman and colleagues in a paper published in the *Archives of Internal Medicine* in September 1983.

The so-called 10 commandments for effective consultations are presented:

1. **Determine the question being asked.**

   As a guiding principle, and when taking the initial phone call from the requesting service, always determine the specific medicine-related question he or she wants answered. This will be helpful, especially in situations in which the patient has an extensive and complicated previous medical history. Thus, a typical consultation note should begin by stating a specific problem, such as "Called to see this 78-year-old woman with type 2 diabetes and hypertension for perioperative glucose control. . . ."

2. **Establish urgency.**

   Always determine if the consult is emergent, urgent, or elective.

3. **Look for yourself.**

   Seldom do the answers to the consultation question lie in the chart; more often than not independent data gathering is required, including reviewing prior admissions. Often the patient requires further testing. In many cases the data review combined with a complete history and physical exam from an internal medicine perspective will establish the diagnosis.

4. **Be as brief as appropriate.**

   It is not necessary to repeat in detail the data already in the primary team's note; obviously as much new data independently gathered should be recorded.

5. **Be specific.**

   Try to be goal-oriented and keep the discussion and differential diagnosis concise. When recommending drugs, always include dose, frequency, and route.

6. **Provide contingency plans.**

   Try to anticipate potential problems (e.g., if using escalating doses of a β-blocker for rapid atrial fibrillation, make sure that regular BP checks are instituted). Staff (nursing/ancillary) on other floors are not used to treating medicine patients.

7. **Honor thy turf.**

   Remember to answer the questions you were asked; it is not appropriate to engage the patient in a detailed discussion of whether surgery is indicated or likely to succeed. In situations in which you are asked by the patient about the surgical procedure, defer to the primary team rather than speculating on the technical aspects of the surgery.

8. **Teach—with tact.**

   Share your insights and expertise without condescension.

9. **Talk is cheap, and effective.**

   Communicate your recommendations directly to the requesting physician. There is no substitute for direct personal contact. Next month the shoe may be on the other foot, and the same resident may be coming to evaluate a surgical abdomen on one of your medicine admissions.

10. **Follow up.**

    Suggestions are more likely to be translated into orders where the consultant continues to follow up.

Preoperative Cardiovascular Risk Assessment

- Preoperative evaluation and intraoperative management are aimed at eliminating or treating risk factors to reduce the risk of cardiac events (MI, unstable angina, CHF, arrhythmia, and death).
- Risk assessment guidelines have recently been suggested by both the American College of Cardiology/American Heart Association Task Force (*J Am Coll Cardiol* 1996;27:910) and the American College of Physicians (*Ann Intern Med* 1997;127:309). Both stress the importance of a thorough clinical assessment with minimal diagnostic testing. History, physical examination, and ECG are important components.
- Patients who have mild CAD on cardiac cath or successful revascularization and have no new clinical symptoms probably have a similar risk for events as patients without CAD.
- The ACP Clinical Guideline and high-risk patient management are detailed in the following two figures.

FIGURE 17-1. Suggested algorithm for the risk assessment and management of patients at low or intermediate risk for perioperative cardiac events. *Risk of irreversible perioperative cardiac events (MI and cardiac death).

FIGURE 17-2. Algorithm for the assessment and management of high-risk patients. AHA, American Heart Association.

- **The Modified Cardiac Risk Index** (*J Gen Intern Med* 1986;1:211) should be performed on all patients (Table 17-1). **Class II or III** predicts a **high risk** for irreversible perioperative cardiac events (MI or cardiac death). **Class I** on the index does not reliably identify those at low risk for perioperative events. The presence of **"low-risk" variables** (*Ann Intern Med* 1989;110:859; and *Am J Cardiol* 1996;77:143) should be determined in these patients (Table 17-2). A substantial number of patients will be at **intermediate risk**. Such patients may benefit from further diagnostic testing, particularly those undergoing vascular surgery.

TABLE 17-1. MODIFIED CARDIAC RISK INDEX

Variable	Points
Coronary artery disease	
MI <6 months earlier	10
MI >6 months earlier	5
Canadian Cardiovascular Society angina classification*	
Class III	10
Class IV	20
Pulmonary edema	
Within 1 week	10
Ever	5
Suspected critical aortic stenosis	20
Arrhythmias	
Rhythm other than NSR or NSR with APCs	5
>5 PVCs on ECG	5
Poor general medical condition, defined as any of the following:	5
PO_2 <60 mm Hg, PCO_2 >50 mm Hg	
K^+ <3 mmol/L, BUN >140 mg/dL	
Creatinine >3 mg/dL	
Bedridden	
Age >70	5
Emergency surgery	10

Class I = 0–15 points
Class II = 20–30 points
Class III >30 points
*Canadian Cardiovascular Society classification of angina: 0 = asymptomatic, I = angina with strenuous exercise, II = angina with moderate exercise, III = angina with walking 1–2 blocks or climbing 1 flight of stairs or less at a normal pace, and IV = inability to perform any physical activity without developing angina.

- β-**Adrenergic antagonists** (Metoprolol, 25 mg PO bid) should be considered in all patients with substantial risk of cardiac disease to reduce mortality and the incidence of cardiovascular complications (*N Engl J Med 1996;335:1713*). If the patient is already taking a β-blocker it should be continued.
- **Nitroglycerin** may be indicated for certain high-risk patients. **Angiotensin-converting enzyme inhibitors and digoxin** should be considered for patients with systolic heart failure. Patients chronically taking a **calcium channel blocker** should continue this medication.

TABLE 17-2. LOW-RISK VARIABLES

Criteria of Eagle et al.*	Criteria of Vanzetto et al.†
Age >70	Age >70
History of angina	History of angina
Diabetes mellitus	Diabetes mellitus
Q wave on ECG	Q wave on ECG
History of ventricular ectopy	History of myocardial infarction
	ST-segment ischemic abnormalities on resting ECG
	Hypertension with severe LVH
	History of CHF

Ann Intern Med 1989;110:859.
†*Am J Cardiol* 1996;77:143.

■ DERMATOLOGY

Toxic Epidermal Necrolysis (TEN)

A. *Emergency—call a consult immediately.*
B. Pertinent information: Drug history. Drugs are nearly always the cause. The most common offenders are sulfonamides, anticonvulsants, penicillin, NSAIDs, and allopurinol.
C. Typical symptoms: Begins with fever, sore throat, burning eyes, 1–3 days before onset of skin involvement.
D. Physical exam findings: High fever, painful erythema of skin with full-thickness epidermal peeling, mucosal and conjunctival erythema.
E. Workup: CBC, blood chemistry profile, CXR, skin biopsy.
F. Diagnosis: Physical exam findings and skin biopsy.
G. Treatment:
   1. Stop suspect drug(s).
   2. Transfer to burn unit/ICU.
   3. IV Fluids, NG tube.
   4. Sterile protocol, antiseptic solution, and nonadherent dressings.

5. Antibiotics only if highly suspicious of sepsis.
6. Consider IVIG.
7. Ophthalmology consult.

H. Clinical pearls: Hepatitis occurs in 10%. Most patients have anemia and lymphopenia. Neutropenia is associated with a poor prognosis. A severe drop in temperature is more indicative of sepsis than fever. Mortality approaches 30% and is most often secondary to sepsis or ARDS. Patients with HIV, systemic lupus, or a bone marrow transplant have a higher risk of developing TEN. SJS is also drug induced and presents with mucosal lesions and less skin involvement. Progression of painful erythema/bullae beyond 10% to 30% of the skin may indicate a transition from SJS to TEN.

Toxic Shock Syndrome

A. *Emergency—call a consult immediately!*

B. Pertinent information: Age of patient, immunocompromised status, menstrual history, postsurgical.

C. Typical signs/symptoms: Painful erythematous skin, sudden onset of high fever, vomiting, diarrhea, sore throat, myalgia, and hypotension.

D. Physical exam: Erythematous scarlatiniform exanthem accentuated on the trunk more than the extremities, progressing to diffuse erythema and edema including the oral mucosa, palms, and soles. Eventually, there is desquamation of the top layer of the epidermis (not full-thickness as in TEN) in 10–12 days.

E. Workup: Blood cultures, CBC, blood chemistry profile, ECG, CXR.

F. Diagnosis: Clinical (fever, typical rash, hypotension, multiorgan involvement).

G. Treatment:
1. Remove any infected foreign bodies.
2. IV antibiotics (penicillinase-resistant anti-*Staphylococcus*).
3. IV fluids.
4. Consider IVIG.
5. Monitor for hypotension/shock.

H. Clinical pearls: *Staphylococcus* scalded skin syndrome has a similar clinical picture; however, it occurs in immunocompromised adults. *S. aureus* is the most common cause of TSS; however, exotoxin-producing streptococci can induce a similar clinical picture associated with higher mortality.

Necrotizing Fasciitis

A. *Emergency—call a surgeon now.*

B. Pertinent info: Recent surgical or traumatic wound.

C. Typical signs and symptoms: Involved area becomes erythematous, indurated, and severely painful. Within hours it can become dusky blue to black, indicating necrosis. Crepitus can develop because of subcutaneous gas formation.

D. Workup and diagnosis: Culture and sensitivity of wound aspirate, plain x-ray for soft tissue gas, and CT/MRI if clinical diagnosis not obvious or to delineate depth of infection.

E. Treatment:
1. Wide surgical debridement
2. IV antibiotics effective against gram-negative bacilli, streptococci, and anaerobes

F. Clinical pearls: Time is essential.

Pemphigus Vulgaris (PV) and Bullous Pemphigoid (BP)

A. Urgent consult.

B. Pertinent info: Flaccid or tense bullae, percentage body involved, mucosal involvement.

C. Typical signs and symptoms: Flaccid bullae with mucosal involvement (PV) and pruritus with tense bullae in an elderly person (BP).

D. Workup and diagnosis: Skin biopsy with direct immunofluorescence and serum for indirect immunofluorescence.

E. Treatment:
1. PV: Prednisone, azathioprine, mycophenolate mofetil, gold.
2. BP: Steroids (topical > systemic), tetracycline, nicotinamide.

F. Clinical pearls: PV is associated with a higher mortality than BP. Thus, PV requires aggressive treatment. Most patients do not require hospitalization unless infected or having difficulty maintaining fluid intake. Causes of blistering diseases include infectious, autoimmune, allergic hypersensitivity, metabolic, and genetic.

Vasculitis

A. Urgent consult.

B. Pertinent info: Drug history, known connective tissue disease, malignancy, or infection.

C. Typical skin findings: Palpable purpura (dark reddish-brown lesions that do not blanch and may blister or ulcerate) on the lower extremities or dependent areas.

D. Workup: CBC, blood chemistry profile, urinalysis, Hemoccult, skin biopsy, CXR, throat culture for strep, ESR, hepatitis panel, cryoglobulins, ANA, RF, antiphospholipid, ANCA, SPEP.

E. Diagnosis: Skin biopsy; concern for systemic involvement if fever, arthralgias, abdominal pain, pulmonary symptoms, hematuria, or proteinuria.

F. Treatment:
1. Discontinue potential causative drug (ASA, sulfonamides, penicillin, barbiturates, amphetamines, PTU).
2. Treat underlying disorder (infection, malignancy, or connective tissue disease).

3. Antihistamines, NSAIDs, colchicine, dapsone, antimalarials.
4. If systemic involvement: Prednisone, azathioprine, cyclophosphamide, IVIG, plasmapheresis.

G. Clinical pearls: 50% of cases are idiopathic. Thrombocytopenia is associated with nonpalpable purpura. DIC and coumadin necrosis cause extensive purpura. *Neisseria* sepsis and Rocky Mountain spotted fever also cause petechiae and purpura. Acral hemorrhagic papules, pustules, or vesicles may result from septic emboli.

Hypersensitivity Syndrome (Severe Drug Reaction)

A. Urgent consult.
B. Pertinent information: Drug history (sulfonamides, anticonvulsants, allopurinol).
C. Physical exam: Maculopapular blanching eruption, exfoliative dermatitis, or erythema multiforme-like lesions mostly on the trunk and proximal extremities, fever, lymphadenopathy, hepatosplenomegaly.
D. Workup: CBC, liver function panel, urinalysis, CXR.
E. Treatment:
   1. Stop drug
   2. Oral steroids
   3. Antihistamines
F. Clinical pearls: The syndrome develops within 8 weeks of starting the causative drug. Up to 50% develop fulminant hepatic necrosis if the drug is not stopped early in the course. Some anticonvulsants cross-react in 70% to 80% of patients (phenytoin, carbamazepine, and phenobarbital). Patients should warn first-degree relatives that they, too, may be at high risk for a reaction to these anticonvulsants.

Erythroderma

A. Urgent consult.
B. Pertinent info: Prior skin disorder, drug history, duration of erythroderma.
C. Physical exam: Diffuse erythema of skin leading to exfoliative dermatitis, pruritus, keratoderma, shivering/chills, alopecia.
D. Labs: CBC, blood chemistry panel, albumin, calcium, SPEP, peripheral blood smear for Sézary cells.
E. Diagnosis: Clinical, skin biopsy.
F. Treatment:
   1. Treat underlying skin condition if known (psoriasis, eczema, etc.).
   2. Discontinue suspect drugs if any.
   3. Search for and treat underlying malignancy.
   4. Topical steroid ointment (midpotency), emollients, systemic antihistamines.
   5. Monitor closely for electrolyte and fluid imbalances, high-output cardiac failure, renal failure, sepsis, and hypothermia.

G. Clinical pearls: 20% of cases are idiopathic. The course and prognosis depend on the underlying etiology. A diligent search for the underlying cause is often required. Most patients do not require hospitalization unless infected or in high-output cardiac failure.

■ NEUROLOGY
Stroke

A. If stroke is suspected, the level of urgency is guided by the time of onset. *If the neurologic deficit occurred within several hours and is persisting or worsening, call a consultation immediately.*

TIAs (ischemic deficits that clear in less than 24 hours, usually within 5–10 minutes) require urgent consultation and attention.

B. General points:
1. When to suspect this:
   a. An acute neurologic deficit that falls within a cerebral vascular territory.
   b. A neurologic deficit involving the loss of speech, cognition, movement, sensation, and vision.
2. What isn't a stroke:
   a. Noncirculatory neurologic problems that appear suddenly or may be noticed relatively acutely that on further questioning reveal themselves to be subacute or chronic.
   b. Positive neurologic symptoms such as pain are unusual.
   c. Syncope, seizure with postictal (Todd's) paralysis, isolated dizziness, memory loss, and confusion (rule out aphasia) have all been mistaken for strokes.
3. Classification:
   a. Hemorrhage (nontraumatic, intraparenchymal, or subarachnoid)
   b. Ischemic stroke
C. Pertinent information:
1. Time course of symptoms (gradual or sudden?).
2. Exact time of onset. When was the patient last known to be normal?
3. Progression of symptoms: Improving, worsening, or staying the same?
4. Did the patient fall?
5. Associated symptoms? Headache, neck pain, nausea, and vomiting suggest hemorrhagic stroke.
6. What are the contraindications for giving acute thrombolytic therapy?
7. Neurologic, general medical, and recent surgical history.
8. Patient's medications including anticoagulation.
D. Physical exam:
1. Vital signs: Blood pressure, pulse, respirations, and temperature; finger-stick glucose level, oxygen saturation.

2. Signs of head injury.
3. Observe for oral trauma that would suggest an unwitnessed seizure.
4. Cardiopulmonary exam focusing on possible arrhythmia, congestive heart failure, aspiration.
5. Focused neurologic exam.

E. Workup:
1. Stat noncontrast CT of the head to differentiate between a hemorrhagic and an ischemic stroke.
2. Basic studies should be obtained such as an ECG, CXR, fingerstick glucose, CBC, chemistry panel, PT, PTT, and urinalysis.

F. Treatment:
1. Intracerebral hemorrhage
   a. Initial management is directed toward the basic ABCs.
      i. Protect the airway and provide oxygenation.
      ii. Intubation should be considered for anyone with:
         • Decreasing level of consciousness.
         • Signs of brain stem dysfunction.
         • Insufficient ventilation as indicated by hypoxia (Po_2 <60 mm Hg or Pco_2 >50 mm Hg) or obvious risk for aspiration regardless of arterial oxygenation.
   b. Blood pressure management.
      i. Hypertension.
         • Avoid overaggressive treatment of elevated blood pressure.
         • Consider antihypertensive therapy only if mean arterial BP >130 (or systolic BP is >180 mm Hg and diastolic BP >105 mm Hg).
         • Commonly used antihypertensive medications.
            Labetalol, 10–40 mg IV boluses q hour
            Hydralazine, 10–20 mg IV q4–6h
      ii. Treat hypotension (systolic arterial blood pressure below 90 mm Hg or below relative baseline).
         • Volume replenishment with isotonic saline is first line.
         • If hypotension persists after correction of volume deficit, pressors should be considered, especially if systolic pressure is <90 mm Hg.
         • Commonly used pressors.
            Phenylephrine, 2–10 μg/kg/min
            Dopamine, 2–20 μg/kg/min
            Norepinephrine, 0.05–0.2 μg/kg/min

2. Ischemic stroke
   a. **Thrombolytic Treatment: Time is Brain!** The only FDA-approved treatment for acute ischemic stroke is thrombolytic therapy, which must be given within 3 hours from time of onset before the risk of symptomatic hemor-

rhage exceeds the benefit of thrombolysis. *Obtain an immediate consultation if you think the patient may qualify for treatment with thrombolytic therapy.*

   b. Blood pressure management.

      i. In practice, treatment is less aggressive in ischemic stroke.

      ii. Consider only if systolic BP is >185 mm Hg or diastolic BP >115 mm Hg, especially if thrombolytic medication is considered or in the presence of other hypertensive crises.

      iii. Treat hypotension.

Seizures

A. Level of urgency/emergency:

- *Status epilepticus is an emergency. Call a consult immediately.*
- New onset of a single seizure requires an immediate assessment into its causes.
- A single seizure recurrence in a patient with a known seizure disorder may need an urgent consult depending on its course and severity.

B. Factors that may influence a more **urgent** consultation:

- Failure to regain cognition and function after the seizure.
- Seizure type or severity atypical for the patient.

C. Important historical information:

- Has mental status returned?
- Describe the seizure:

      a. Describe the movements (rhythmic, asynchronous, one side involved more than the other, head turning left or right).

- Known seizure disorder?
- Known metabolic disorder?

D. Physical exam:

Signs of head injury, oropharyngeal trauma, signs of meningismus, arrhythmia, occurrence of aspiration, neurologic exam with focus on the level of consciousness, any focal signs of cranial nerve impairment and motor or sensory loss.

E. Workup information:

1. A seizure is a symptom; search for an etiology (consider structural causes, infections, stroke, trauma, metabolic, iatrogenic, neoplastic).
2. Labs include Accucheck, Na, Ca, Mg, Phos, and BUN/Cr.

F. Treatment:

1. What to do when a patient is having a seizure:

      a. Remain calm. Determine if the patient is still having a seizure.

      b. Take measures to protect the patient.

         i. Place the patient in the lateral decubitus position with suctioning nearby.

    ii. Pad the bed rails to avoid head injury.

    iii. Remove sharp and hard objects that may potentially cause injury.

  c. Attend to the ABCs.

    i. Provide oxygen by cannula or nonrebreather face mask.

    ii. Protect the airway.

    iii. Obtain vital signs.

    iv. Obtain a finger-stick glucose.

2. If the patient is still having seizures, either continuous activity lasting >5 minutes or two or more discrete seizures between which there is incomplete recovery of consciousness, status epilepticus has developed. Note that two seizures between which there is recovery of consciousness does not define status.

Status Epilepticus

A. *Emergency—call a consult immediately!*

B. Definition: Continuous seizure for >5 minutes or two or more discrete seizures with incomplete recovery of consciousness.

C. Treatment:

1. Ensure adequate respiration (100% O_2 by mask); have airway box/suction at bedside available; have intubation kit ready.

2. Establish ECG monitor, continuous pulse oximetry, and ABG.

3. NG tube placement.

4. Obtain vitals including temperature.

5. Ensure IV access.

6. Labs: Obtain glucose stick, serum chemistries including Na, Ca, Mg, phos, urine tox, serum tox, ETOH, UA, drug levels, and CBC.

7. Give 50 mL of 50% glucose with thiamine, 100 mg IVP. Untreated hypoglycemia has much more serious consequences than transient hyperglycemia.

8. Administer lorazepam (Ativan), 0.1 mg/kg IV (4–8 mg at a maximum of 2 mg/min); if no IV access, rectal diazepam, 0.5 mg/kg.

9. Phenytoin IV, 15–20 mg/kg (in dextrose-free solution) at a rate of 1 mg/kg/min to a maximum of 50 mg/min (monitor BP and cardiac rhythm). Alternatively, fosphenytoin can be used. It tends to be safer with less risk of hypotension.

10. **Persistent refractory status:** If seizures continue >60 minutes.

  a. Intubation and transfer to an ICU with continuous EEG monitoring.

  b. Pentobarbital, 5–12 mg/kg bolus then infusion 1.5 mg/kg/hr increased q5–10min until status stopped or flat EEG obtained.

     c. Midazolam, 0.2 mg/kg IV bolus then 0.1–0.6 mg/kg/hr: Induces less hypotension and cardiorespiratory depression and can be easily titrated; however, tachyphylaxis is a problem.

     d. Propofol, 3–5 mg/kg bolus, then infusion at 1–15 mg/kg/hr.

11. When IV access is not available:

     a. Rectal diazepam at 0.5 mg/kg (maximum 20 mg).

     b. Intramuscular midazolam, 0.2 mg/kg bolus (mean time to peak serum concentration 25 minutes).

     c. Intranasal midazolam; usually terminates within 10 minutes of administration (0.15–0.3 mg/kg).

D. Clinical pearls:

1. Treat the underlying cause and optimize dose of medications.

2. Urine dipstick to detect myoglobin to watch for rhabdomyolysis.

3. Treat hyperthermia (40°C core) with a cooling blanket, antipyretics.

Bacterial Meningitis

A. Level of urgency/emergency. When suspected, urgent evaluation is required for prompt diagnosis and treatment, and can minimize the neurologic complications following acute bacterial meningitis.

B. When to suspect this:

- History of myalgias, ear pain, sore throat, joint stiffness, fatigue occurring several days before major clinical deterioration is often noted.

- Fever and vomiting are the most consistent early signs, present in more than three-fourths of patients.

- Headache, often described as bursting and splitting, is severe enough to overcome the most commonly prescribed medications. Photophobia may be present.

- Altered level of consciousness occurs in most patients, varying from delirium to drowsiness and stupor. An acute confusional state in a febrile elderly patient, for example, should always raise the possibility of acute bacterial meningitis and should not be assumed to have resulted from a pneumonia or urinary tract infection.

C. Physical exam:

1. Seizures may develop at some point in the course of the disease.

2. Careful neurologic exam is essential. Flexion of the neck that results in spontaneous flexion of the knees (Brudzinski's sign) and passive extension of the knees while the hips are flexed results in eye opening and a verbal response (Kernig's sign).

3. Papilledema may suggest superior sagittal sinus thrombosis or progressive brain edema.

4. Rash (petechial or purpuric) suggests *Neisseria meningitidis*, less often *Staphylococcus aureus*, pneumococcus, or rickettsiae.

D. Workup:
  1. Blood cultures and urgent lumbar puncture are required.
  2. Obtain a head CT before LP to rule out a mass effect as a cause of the altered level of consciousness, especially if there is a finding of focality or increased intracranial pressure.
  3. When CT cannot be done in a timely fashion, blood cultures should be obtained and empiric antibiotic therapy started. CT should then be performed followed by urgent LP afterward.

TABLE 17-3. CSF ANALYSIS

Condition	Color	Pressure (mm H$_2$O)	Cells (No./mL)	Protein (mg/dL)	Glucose (mg/dL)
Normal	Clear	70–180	0–5 mononu-clear	15–45	45–80 (two-thirds of serum glucose)
Bacterial meningitis	Opales-cent	Increased (may be normal)	>5 to many 1,000 PMNs	50–1,500	0–45
Viral infection	Clear or opales-cent	Normal (may be slightly increased)	>5–2,000, mostly lymphs	20–200	Normal (may be slightly decreased)
Tuberculous men-ingitis	Clear or opales-cent	Increased (may be normal)	>5–500 lymphs	45–500	10–45
Fungal meningitis	Clear or opales-cent	Normal or increased	>5–800 lymphs	Normal or increased	Normal or decreased
Carcino-matous meningitis	Clear or opales-cent	Normal or increased	>5–1,000 mononu-clear	Up to 500	Normal or decreased
Subarach-noid hem-orrhage	Bloody or xantho-chromic	Increased (may be normal)	Many RBC; ratio of WBC/RBC same as blood	Up to 2,000	Normal

TABLE 17-4. TREATMENT OPTIONS

Age or Clinical Setting	Likely Organism	Empiric Treatment
Immunocompetent		
18–50 years	*Staphylococcus pneumoniae, Neisseria meningitidis*	Broad-spectrum cephalosporin
>50 years	*S. pneumoniae, L. monocytogenes*, gram-negative bacilli	Broad-spectrum cephalosporin + ampicillin
TB	*Mycobacterium tuberculosis*	Isoniazid + rifampin + ethambutol + pyrazinamide
Head trauma, CSF shunt, neurosurgery	Staphylococci, gram-negative bacilli, *S. pneumoniae*	Vancomycin + ceftazidime
Immunocompromised	*L. monocytogenes*, gram-negative bacilli, also *S. pneumoniae* and *Haemophilus influenzae*	Ampicillin + ceftazidime

Viral Infections

A. This is an urgent consultation. Prognosis depends on rapid diagnosis and stage of the illness when treatment is begun.

B. Symptoms: Altered consciousness, fever, change in personality, headache, a flu-like illness may precede initial symptoms by a few days.

C. Physical exam: Assess mental status, focusing on level of consciousness, language, and memory. Look for signs of autonomic dysfunction.

D. Diagnosis:
   1. Once HSV is suspected, start acyclovir (see Treatment section) while diagnostic studies are pending.
   2. MRI: More sensitive than CT and is therefore the first choice. T2 hyperintensity of the temporal and orbitofrontal lobes may be present.
   3. CT may be normal early or show signs of low attenuation in the anterior and mesial temporal lobes.
   4. CSF studies: Do not do LP if evidence of mass effect.
      CSF is normal in 5% to 10% of cases. Refer to Table 17-3 for more information.
      CSF PCR: Highly sensitive (95%) and specific; remains positive up to 5 days after starting acyclovir.
   5. EEG: Usually abnormal.

E. Treatment:
   1. Acyclovir: 10 mg/kg IV q8 × 10–14 days if diagnosis is confirmed. Monitor and follow renal function closely in patients with renal impairment.

2. If a temporal lobe lesion typical of HSV is present along with edema on head imaging, reduce ICP (20 mg bolus of dexamethasone IV, then 4 mg q4h). If mass effect produces a midline shift >3 mm or the patient deteriorates or is comatose, intubate, and hyperventilate to a P_{CO_2} of 28–30 mm Hg. If herniation is impending, IV mannitol, 50–100 g, should be given.

F. Clinical pearls:
   1. Prompt recognition and treatment of suspected cases minimizes neurologic complications.
   2. HSV encephalitis makes up approximately 10% to 20% of adult cases of acute encephalitis.
   3. Positive predictors of bacterial meningitis (99% PPV)
      - Glucose <34 mg/dL
      - Protein >200 mg/dL
      - CSF/serum glucose <0.23
      - WBC >2,000/mm^3
      - PMNs >1,180/mm^3.

Neuroleptic Malignant Syndrome

A. Urgent consult.
B. When to suspect:
   1. May arise during early treatment with neuroleptic therapy, most often when doses are increased quickly or from a previously well-tolerated neuroleptic.
   2. Dehydration and hyponatremia may be predisposing factors.
   3. Has the patient been on other medications such as selective serotonin reuptake inhibitors, tetrabenazine, or acutely withdrawn from an antiparkinsonian medication?
C. History and physical exam: Fever, extreme rigidity, dysautonomia, depressed level of consciousness, tremor, dystonia, and other dyskinesias are prominent.
D. Workup:
   1. Diagnosis is primarily by history.
   2. An elevated CK level is nonspecific but may help with the diagnosis.
   3. Other considerations include meningitis, encephalitis, systemic infection, heat stroke, and malignant hyperthermia.
E. Treatment:
   1. Withdraw the neuroleptic immediately.
   2. Mortality results from complications of hyperthermia.
   3. Treat hyperthermia aggressively with antipyretics and cooling blanket.
   4. Consider dantrolene (1–2 mg/kg IV up to 10 mg/kg maximum), followed by 4–8 mg/kg in four divided doses per day for 3 days.
   5. Monitor frequently for autonomic dysfunction.
   6. Manage fluid status and electrolytes.

■ OBSTETRICS AND GYNECOLOGY

Key Points

A. Obtain a menstrual history including LMP, pregnancy status, age at menarche, duration between menses, length of menses, amount of vaginal bleeding (i.e., how many pads soaked in how many hours?).

B. Also ask about last Pap smear, history of abnormal Pap smear results, history of any postmenopausal bleeding.

C. Obtain an obstetric history: Gravida and para status (including full-term deliveries, premature deliveries, stillbirths, abortions or miscarriages, and living children).

D. Obtain a sexual history including form of contraception, number of partners, bleeding with intercourse, and history of sexually transmitted diseases.

E. Perform a physical exam including a pelvic exam. If access to a speculum or pelvic table is limited, then a bimanual and rectovaginal exam can be performed at the bedside.

Ectopic Pregnancy

A. *Emergency—call a consult immediately!*

B. History: Date of patient's LMP, menstrual history, type of contraception (if any), history of tubal ligation, history of ectopic pregnancy, amount of vaginal bleeding (if any), and degree of abdominal pain (if any).

C. Physical exam: Take **vital signs immediately** with orthostatics and fetal heart tones auscultated by Doppler.

D. Workup: Tests to be drawn include CBC, type and screen, and urine pregnancy test (if positive, draw a quantitative β-hCG immediately). Note: History of a tubal ligation does not by any means rule out an ectopic pregnancy.

E. Treatment:
  1. Place large-bore IV immediately.
  2. The gynecologic consult team should be notified **immediately** if:
     - Pregnancy test result is positive
     - No fetal heart tones are heard
     - History of vaginal bleeding or abdominal pain.
  3. If there is a positive pregnancy test result and hemodynamic instability exists, resuscitation with blood and prompt surgical exploration is necessary.

Vaginal Bleeding

A. *Heavy vaginal bleeding can be an emergency—call a consult immediately!*

B. History:
  - Assess how long the bleeding has lasted, where the patient is in her cycle, how much bleeding has occurred, if there is a history of bleeding disorders, and whether the patient is on hormones, contraception, or anticoagulants, and when she last took any of these medications or if any of the medication

has been recently changed. Determine by history whether the bleeding is chronic or acute.

Type and cross the patient if the bleeding is heavy, the patient is unstable, or both, and make sure a pregnancy test has been done and large-bore IV has been placed.

- Assess risk factors for cervical cancer (history of abnormal Pap smear results, smoking, multiparity, low socioeconomic group, number of sexual partners, age at first intercourse, history of cervical cancer).
- Assess risk factors for endometrial cancer (obesity, diabetes, hypertension, unopposed estrogen consumption, history of abnormal endometrial biopsies, early age at menarche or late age at menopause, history of anovulation, family history of endometrial cancer or history of colon or breast cancer).

C. Physical exam: Determine source of bleeding—make sure the bleeding is from the vagina or uterus and not the urethra (inspect the urethra), bladder (do a straight catheterization), or rectum (rectal exam).

D. Workup: Pregnancy test (if positive, do a type and screen for Rh status and the need for RhoGAM for **all** patients), CBC.

E. Treatment:
1. Place large-bore IV.
2. Rehydration with fluids; transfuse with pRBC if unstable.
3. D/C any anticoagulants.
4. Notify Ob/Gyn consultant.

Pelvic Mass

A. *Call a gynecology consult immediately for suspected ovarian torsion.* Other causes do not require emergent consultation.

B. History: Obtain a thorough history including menstrual history, menopausal status, pregnancy status, history of neoplasia, history of vaginal bleeding, last Pap smear, history or recent biopsy of any gynecologic organs, and history of any gynecologic surgery. Ask about family history of ovarian, breast, or colon cancer, and history of tobacco use.

C. Physical exam: Perform pelvic exam (including speculum exam) to thoroughly visualize the cervix, bimanual and rectovaginal exam to assess motility, position, and further characterize the mass.

D. Workup: Radiologic exams include abdominal/pelvic CT (determine the position in relation to other pelvic organs [adnexa, uterus, cervix], size of the mass, if the mass is complex, fluid- or blood-filled areas, and whether calcifications are present). Patient may need a pelvic ultrasound.

E. Clinical pearls: The differential diagnosis includes neoplasms and benign cysts but may also involve ovarian torsion. Torsion may present as a pelvic mass but is usually accompanied by intermittent severe abdominal pain, tender pelvic mass by exam, low-grade temperatures, and on pelvic ultrasound may be accompanied by decreased flow to the ovary.

■ **OPHTHALMOLOGY**
Trauma with Possible Ruptured Globe
A. *Ocular emergency—call a consult immediately!*
B. Pertinent information: Age, PMH/PSH/ocular history, allergies, current meds including ocular meds, specific ocular complaints, history of events preceding trauma, specific chemicals or items involved.
C. Typical symptoms: Pain, decreased vision, history of trauma.
D. Physical exam findings: 360-degree subconjunctival heme, full thickness corneal or scleral laceration, irregular pupil, exposed intraocular contents, hyphema.
E. Treatment:
1. Place a shield over the involved eye; **do not touch ocular contents**.
2. NPO (determine last meal).
3. IV antibiotics (i.e., Ancef/Ceftaz/Vanc) 1 gm IV now.
4. Orbital CT scan (axial and coronal).
5. Surgical repair within 24 hours.
F. Clinical pearls:
1. In trauma with eyelid laceration; do NOT try to repair the laceration. Allow ophthalmologist to assess extent.
2. If there is severe eyelid swelling, this is a possible sign of orbital cellulitis.
3. Significant orbital trauma may require evaluation for retrobulbar heme, optic nerve trauma, and fractures.

Injury

Acute Chemical Splash
A. *Ocular emergency—BEGIN IRRIGATION, then call a consult immediately.*
B. Pertinent information: Age, PMH/PSH/ocular history, allergies, current meds including ocular meds, specific ocular complaints, history of events, specific chemicals or items involved, time, irrigation.
C. Symptoms: ± Pain, blurry vision, foreign body sensation, tearing, photophobia.
D. Physical exam:
1. Mild to moderate splash: Sloughing of entire epithelium, hyperemia, mild chemosis, eyelid edema, first or second degree periocular skin burns.
2. Moderate to severe: Pronounced chemosis, perilimbal blanching, corneal edema or opacification, anterior chamber reaction/no view of the anterior chamber, increased intraocular pressure, second or third degree burns.
E. Workup: Slit-lamp exam, evert eyelids, check pH, intraocular pressure.

F. Immediate treatment:
  1. COPIOUS IRRIGATION with 1 L of any available irrigant (e.g., NS, ½ NS, or LR), and keep irrigating until you talk with the consultant.
  2. May give 1–2 drops of topical anesthetic.
  3. Do NOT use acid or alkali to neutralize splash.
  4. Check pH 5 minutes after irrigation.

G. Treatment AFTER irrigation:
  1. Debride necrotic tissue
  2. Topical antibiotic ointment: Polysporin, erythromycin/Ciloxan ophthalmic qid
  3. Cycloplege with homatropine 5% bid (avoid phenylephrine)
  4. Topical steroid: Pred Forte 1% or Pred Mild qid
  5. Pressure patch
  6. Antiglaucoma drops: Timoptic 0.5% or Alphagan 0.2% bid prn
  7. Daily follow-up with ophthalmology, gradual taper of steroids

Corneal Ulcer

A. *This is an emergency—call a consult immediately.*
B. Pertinent information: Age, past ocular history, history leading up to event (recent trauma or contact lens use).
C. Symptoms: Pain, photophobia, decreased vision, ± discharge.
D. Physical exam: Focal opacity/overlying epithelial defect, anterior chamber reaction, hypopyon, eyelid edema.
E. Workup: Gram's stain and fungal culture, *E. coli* overlay.
F. Treatment:
  1. Ocuflox drops, q2–4h, and cycloplege with homatropine 5% bid.
  2. If ulcer is severe: admit and give fortified Ancef, 50 mg/mL, and tobramycin, 15 mg/mL drops q hour.
G. Clinical pearls: Contact lens wearers are at much higher risk. Bacterial, fungal, HSV, and *Acanthamoeba* are all possible causes.

Corneal Abrasion or Foreign Body

A. This is usually not an emergency, but consult if in doubt.
B. Pertinent information: Age, past ocular history, history of events leading up to event, occupational history (i.e., grinding, drilling, trauma), contact lens use, type of foreign body.
C. Symptoms: Acute pain, tearing, photophobia.
D. Workup:
  1. Blue light or slit-lamp exam with fluorescein to detect epithelial irregularities.
  2. Look for foreign body or rust ring.
  3. Measure and record dimension of irregularities.
  4. Evert eyelids to look for hidden foreign bodies.
  5. Look for associated corneal ulcers.

E. Treatment:
   1. Remove foreign body (preferably by an ophthalmologist).
   2. Noncontact lens wearers: Cycloplege with homatropine 5% bid, Polysporin, or erythromycin ointment tid, patch.
   3. Contact lens wearers: NO patch, Ciloxan qid × 7 days.
   4. Follow up next day with an ophthalmologist and close follow-up as needed thereafter.
F. Clinical pearls: If you remove corneal metallic foreign bodies, make sure there is no rust ring left behind. If there is any chance of penetrating injury, call a consult immediately.

Acute Vision Loss

Central Retinal Artery Occlusion

A. *Ocular emergency—call a consult STAT!*
B. Pertinent information: Age, PMH/PSH/ocular history, allergies, current meds including ocular meds, specific ocular complaints, history preceding event, vision loss.
C. Symptoms: Painless, unilateral, acute loss of vision, prior history of amaurosis fugax.
D. Physical exam: Whitening of the retina with a "cherry red" spot in the center of the macula, afferent pupillary defect (Marcus Gunn pupil), narrowed arterioles, occasionally arteriolar emboli/plaque visible.
E. Workup: ESR, fasting BS, CBC, PT/PTT, ANA/RF, RPR/FTA-Ab, check BP, carotid Dopplers, cardiac Echo.
F. Treatment:
   1. Ocular massage (digital or fundus contact lens).
   2. Anti-glaucoma drops (Timoptic, Iopidine, Trusopt, Xalatan, and/or Diamox, 250 mg PO × 2).
   3. Call ophthalmologist again if not present.
G. Clinical pearls: Etiology can be embolic (carotid or cardiac), thrombosis, giant cell arteritis, collagen vascular disease, hypercoagulable disorders (i.e., SLE, PAN), retinal detachment, or rare causes (i.e., migraines, Behçet's syndrome, syphilis).

Acute Angle-Closure Glaucoma

A. *Ocular emergency—call consult immediately!*
B. Pertinent information: Age, PMH/PSH/ocular history, allergies, current meds including ocular meds, specific ocular complaints, family history, recent surgery, recent laser surgery.
C. Symptoms: Pain, blurry vision, colored halos around lights, frontal headache, n/v.
D. Physical exam: Beefy red conjunctival injection, fixed, mid-dilated pupil (usually in one eye), shallow anterior chamber, acutely elevated intraocular pressure (40s or above!).
E. Workup: Slit-lamp exam, measure intraocular pressure.

F. Treatment:
   1. Topical anti-glaucoma drops (Timoptic, Alphagan, Trusopt, Xalatan).
   2. Topical steroid Pred Forte 1% (q15min × 4 doses).
   3. Carbonic anhydrase inhibitor IV or PO (i.e., Diamox 250 mg IV or sorbitol 100 g PO).
   4. Osmotic agent (isosorbide, mannitol).
   5. Phakic (pilocarpine 1–2%), aphakic (cycloplege).
   6. Definitive (laser) treatment by ophthalmologist.
G. Clinical pearls: Be aware of patient's cardiovascular and pulmonary status, evaluate electrolyte/renal status before starting carbonic anhydrase inhibitors or osmotic agents. Etiology can be from an anatomic pupillary block, neovascular, anterior displacement of lens-iris diaphragm (i.e., choroidals, tumor), malignant glaucoma, medications (i.e., mydriatics, anticholinergics).

Papilledema (Disc Edema Secondary to Increased Intracranial Pressure)

A. *Ocular emergency—call a consult immediately!*
B. Pertinent information: Age, PMH/PSH/ocular history, allergies, current meds including ocular meds, specific ocular complaints, history of events preceding trauma.
C. Symptoms: Transient vision loss, headache, n/v, diplopia, scotomata.
D. Physical exam: Bilateral swollen, hyperemic discs, blurring of disc margins, obscured vessels, cotton-wool spots, dilated/tortuous veins, normal pupillary response, and color vision.
E. Workup: Check BP, careful ocular exam (pupils, color vision, exam of fundus), urgent orbit, and head CT. Neurology consult and consider LP, CBC, TSH, ESR.
F. Treatment:
   1. Treat underlying cause!
G. Clinical pearls: Etiologies you may see on a medical service include pseudotumor cerebri, subdural/subarachnoid hemorrhage, AVM or sagittal sinus thrombosis, intracranial tumors, brain abscess, meningitis/encephalitis, hydrocephalus, malignant HTN, uveitis, infiltrative disease (i.e., sarcoid, TB, syphilis), ischemic optic neuropathy (i.e., giant cell arteritis), central retinal vein occlusion, papillitis (i.e., multiple sclerosis/optic neuritis, diabetic eye disease). It is often helpful to communicate the level of confidence of your fundus exam to the consultant.

Retinal Detachment

A. *Ocular urgency—call a consult.*
B. Pertinent information: Age, PMH/PSH/ocular history, allergies, current meds, specific complaints, history of preceding trauma or surgery.
C. Symptoms: Painless unilateral decreased vision with associated flashes and floaters, curtain or veil across vision, relative visual field defect.

D. Physical exam: typically a "white & quiet"–appearing eye—externally looks normal, usually NO afferent pupillary defect unless a large retinal detachment. Fundus exam reveals a white, billowing, or wrinkled retina.

E. Workup: Slit-lamp exam and dilated fundus exam.

F. Treatment:
  1. No acute intervention
  2. Low level activity
  3. Needs a retina specialist evaluation

G. Clinical pearls: Risk factors include recent eye surgery, ocular trauma, high myopia, and a retinal detachment in contralateral eye. A peripheral retinal tear or hole may present with only flashes or floaters and no change in vision. These still require urgent ophthalmologic intervention.

Infection

Endophthalmitis (Infection of the Inside of the Eye)

A. *Ocular emergency—call a consult immediately!*

B. Pertinent information: Age, PMH/PSH/ocular history, allergies, current meds including ocular meds, history of ocular surgery or trauma.

C. Symptoms: Unilateral painful eye, decreased vision.

D. Physical exam: Moderate injection, hypopyon (pus behind the cornea), poor red reflex or view to the back of the eye.

E. Treatment:
  1. Emergent ophthalmologic evaluation
  2. Admission
  3. IV vancomycin or Ancef 1 gm q12h + Ceftaz 1 gm q12h
  4. May need culture and injected antibiotics

F. Clinical pearls: A diagnosis of endophthalmitis must be considered FIRST in any patient with recent ocular surgery!

Herpes Simplex

A. This is not an ocular emergency, but urgent referral to ophthalmologist is strongly recommended.

B. Pertinent information: Age, PMH, ocular history, possible mode of transmission.

C. Symptoms: Usually unilateral, pain, tearing, photophobia.

D. Physical exam: Skin vesicles, conjunctival injection and follicles, dendritic keratitis, iritis, uveitis, retinitis.

E. Treatment:
  1. Viroptic 1% or Vira A ointment 5×/day for 7 days.
  2. Acyclovir, 200 mg PO 5×/day or Valtrex, 500 mg PO tid.
  3. Homatropine 5% drops bid.
  4. Pred Forte 1% drops qid (do NOT give steroids with epithelial disease).
  5. Empiric coverage with Polysporin drops qid is recommended.
  6. Follow up next day with ophthalmologist.

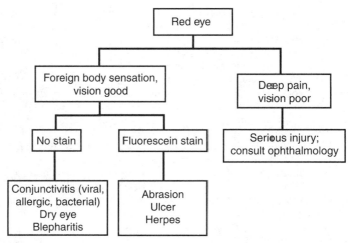

FIGURE 17-3. The red eye.

The Red Eye

Conjunctivitis

A. This is not an emergency.

B. Pertinent information: Age, possible contacts, past ocular history, allergies or previous history of allergic conjunctivitis, make sure there is no pain involved for allergic and viral conjunctivitis.

C. Symptoms:
Viral: Unilateral red eye, possible associated URI symptoms, mild itching, morning crusting or discharge.
Allergic: Bilateral itching, mild redness, watery discharge.
Bacterial: Acute purulent discharge, eyelid edema, decreased vision.

D. Physical exam:
Viral: Conjunctival injection, crusting, follicles.
Allergic: Lid swelling, chemosis, papillae.
Bacterial: Discharge.

E. Workup:
Bacterial: Gram's stain and culture for *staphylococcus*, *Streptococcus*, *H. flu*, GC.

F. Treatment:
Viral:
1. No specific medical treatment necessary—self-limited illness.
2. Symptomatic treatment with cool compresses or artificial tears.
3. Naphcon A or Vasocon may be prescribed tid ×7 days.
4. Wash hands, towels, pillowcases. Use separate towels. No contact lens wear for at least 7 days.

    5. Avoid close contact (especially rubbing eyes and touching others) without washing hands first.

    Allergic:

    1. Eliminate inciting agent.

    2. Cool compresses and artificial tears.

    3. Patanol or Allocril antihistamine drops bid.

    Bacterial:

    1. Polysporin ophthalmic ointment or erythromycin ointment qid.

    2. For *H. flu*: Augmentin, 250–500 tid.

    3. For GC: Ceftriaxone, 1 gm IM, and empiric treatment for chlamydia. Treat sexual partners.

G. Clinical pearls: If vision is acutely and significantly reduced, a diagnosis of conjunctivitis is UNLIKELY. Any pupillary inequality in a patient with red eye(s) is a danger signal for serious ocular disease.

Acute Hordeolum (Stye)

A. Not an emergency.

B. Symptoms: Pain, redness, "bump."

C. Physical exam: Red, tender, swollen nodule around the lid margin or hair follicle.

D. Treatment:

    1. Hot compress to eyelids for 5 minutes 5×/day.

    2. Empiric topical antibiotic. Polysporin or erythromycin ophthalmic ointment tid.

    3. Follow up with ophthalmologist in 1 week.

■ ORTHOPEDIC SURGERY

Fractures

A. *Open fractures and fractures with associated neurovascular compromise are emergencies—call a consult immediately!*

B. Pertinent history: Mechanism of injury and preinjury level of activity.

C. Pertinent physical exam: Complete distal neurologic and vascular exam.

D. Before calling an orthopedic consult for fracture, plain radiographs of the bone involved must be obtained. Usually AP and lateral views are sufficient. However, in certain instances additional views are necessary. The following list contains some common fractures in which additional views are necessary for diagnosis, preop planning, or both.

    1. Shoulder/proximal humerus: AP, true AP, axillary view, scapular lateral (or Y) view.

    2. Femoral neck/intertrochanteric fractures: AP hip, cross-table lateral, AP ortho pelvis.

    3. Acetabular fractures: AP ortho pelvis, Judet views.

    4. Ankle: AP, lateral, mortise.

    5. Foot: AP, lateral, medial oblique; obtain a Harris heel (axial) view if a calcaneal fracture is suspected.

E. Describing fractures: Attempt to delineate the following:
    1. Fracture pattern (transverse, oblique, spiral)
    2. Displacement
    3. Angulation
    4. Shortening
    5. Comminution
    6. Open versus closed:
      • Open fractures are graded I–III, with III being most severe.
      • Grade I fractures have wounds less than 1 cm in length.
      • Grade II fractures have wounds greater than 1 cm.
      • Grade III fractures are subdivided as follows:
        IIIa: Wound >10 cm without periosteal stripping
        IIIb: Periosteal stripping
        IIIc: Associated vascular injury.

F. Workup: Usually plain radiographs are sufficient. However, if an occult fracture is suspected, obtain either an MRI or a bone scan to confirm. For hip fractures, bone scans may not be positive until 2–3 days postinjury. MRI will be positive within 24 hours.

G. Initial treatment/management:
    1. Open fractures require emergent operative debridement and fixation.
    2. Keep patients NPO.
    3. Give tetanus toxoid.
    4. Give IV antibiotics according to fracture grade.
      • Grade I fractures—cefazolin
      • Grade II fractures—cefazolin and gentamicin
      • Grade III fractures—cefazolin, gentamicin, and penicillin (if associated with gross soft tissue contamination)
    5. Closed fractures are treated on an individual basis based on particular bone involvement and amount of displacement.
    6. When lower extremity fractures are diagnosed, consider initiating DVT prophylaxis with antiembolism stockings and sequential compressive devices, subcutaneous low-molecular-weight heparin, or both.

Septic Joint

A. *This is an **emergency**—call a consult immediately!*

B. Pertinent information: history and exam consistent with effusion, warmth, painful range of motion, tenderness, and fever.

C. Workup: plain radiographs, CBC, ESR, CRP, and blood cultures (if febrile). The diagnosis is confirmed with joint aspiration. Aspiration may be done by the primary physician or an orthopedics consultant. Synovial fluid should be sent for stat Gram's stain, cell count, crystals, and culture. Antibiotics should not be administered until a joint aspirate is obtained.

The patient should be made NPO until the cell count and Gram's stain result are found to be negative for sepsis.

D. Diagnosis:
1. Septic arthritis is diagnosed with a synovial fluid leukocyte count generally >80,000 per cubic mm, a positive Gram's stain, or a positive culture result.
2. An inflammatory/autoimmune arthropathy typically has a synovial fluid leukocyte count of 10,000–50,000 per cubic mm with positive crystals (for gout or CPPD disease), and negative Gram's stain and culture results.

E. Treatment:
1. Operative drainage. [*Neisseria* species (*gonorrhoeae* and *meningitidis*) are exceptions to this rule, as they are highly responsive to antibiotic therapy; operative debridement is not necessary.]
2. Appropriate intravenous antibiotics as determined by cultures. The course of antibiotics is typically 6 weeks total with the first 1–2 weeks being intravenous antibiotics.
3. Once the diagnosis is confirmed, the patient should be made NPO in preparation for operative drainage.

F. Clinical pearls: *S. aureus* is the most common orthopedic pathogen overall. In sexually active adolescents and adults, *N. gonorrhoeae* has a particularly high prevalence, whereas *Salmonella* has a particularly high prevalence in sickle cell patients.

Compartment Syndrome

A. *Compartment syndrome is an emergency. Call the orthopedics consultant emergently.*
B. Definition: Compartment syndromes are caused by elevated hydrostatic pressure within a fascial compartment, leading to tissue ischemia as compartment pressure exceeds capillary pressure. Elevated hydrostatic pressure commonly occurs from bleeding or swelling from within the compartment.
C. When to consider this: The most specific signs and symptoms of compartment syndrome are pain out of proportion to injury, pain with passive stretch of the muscles in the involved compartment, and hard tense compartments. Paraesthesias, pallor, pulselessness, and paralysis may or may not be present. All external circumferential dressings should be removed before examining a patient for compartment syndrome.

Typical history may include the following:
1. Trauma (fracture or muscle contusion)
2. Ischemia
3. Venous obstruction
4. Massive inflammation from snake/insect bites
5. Bleeding into the compartment (consider in anticoagulated patients)

    6. Infiltration of fluid material into a compartment (paint gun injuries)

    7. Tight circumferential dressings

D. Diagnosis: The diagnosis is a clinical one. However, when clinical signs are equivocal, compartment pressures may be measured by an orthopedics consultant. Compartment pressures >30 mm Hg (or a diastolic blood pressure compartment pressure difference >30 mm Hg for hypotensive patients) are diagnostic for compartment syndrome.

E. Treatment:

    1. Make patient NPO immediately.

    2. Emergent fasciotomy.

F. Clinical pearls: Remember that myoglobinuria can occur with compartment syndrome from muscle necrosis.

Acute Cauda Equina Syndrome

A. *This is an emergency—call a consult immediately!*

B. Definition: Cauda equina syndrome is an injury to the spinal canal located between the conus and the lumbosacral nerve roots, resulting in bowel and bladder dysfunction, saddle anesthesia, severe lower extremity neurologic deficit, and anal sphincter laxity.

C. Pertinent history: Suspect in a patient with low back pain and the previously mentioned signs and symptoms.

D. Pertinent physical exam: A complete lower extremity neurologic exam should be performed including lower extremity strength, sensation, and reflexes. A rectal exam should also be performed to assess rectal tone and perianal sensation. Remember that the cauda equina functions as the peripheral nervous system. Therefore, in a complete cauda equina injury, all peripheral nerves to the bowel, bladder, perianal area, and lower extremities will be lost, resulting in absent bulbocavernosus, anal wink, and lower extremity reflexes.

E. Workup: Stat AP and lateral views of the lumbar spine and a stat MRI of the lumbar spine. If the patient has had a prior discectomy, obtain MRI with gadolinium contrast. If the patient has had previous spine instrumentation, obtain a CT myelogram.

F. Treatment:

    1. Make patient NPO immediately.

    2. Emergent operative decompression.

■ OTOLARYNGOLOGY

Airway Emergencies

A. *Call a consult or the airway pager immediately for assistance!*

B. Pertinent history: When the stridor commenced; how long has it persisted; is it constant or intermittent; and is it progressing and to what degree (the degree of stridor may not necessarily indicate the severity of obstruction)? History of prior intubation (and any previous difficulty); trauma; laryngeal surgery; or previous tracheostomy?

C. Pertinent physical exam: Cardinal sign of airway obstruction is stridor secondary to turbulence of air in the upper airways. Inspiratory stridor usually demonstrates partial supraglottic obstruction (i.e., trauma/fractures, foreign bodies, hematomas, edema). Expiratory stridor usually demonstrates glottic or subglottic pathology. Combined inspiratory and expiratory stridor suggests partial obstruction at the level of the glottis. Other signs of respiratory distress may include restlessness, drooling, suprasternal retractions, and hoarseness. A hoarse voice may mean laryngeal involvement. A muffled cry may mean supraglottic involvement. Coughing or choking may refer to vocal cord paralysis, aspiration, reflux, or an anatomic abnormality (laryngeal cleft or TE fistula).

D. Workup: Usually in a true emergent airway, there is no time for diagnostic tests until a stable airway is attained. Some diagnostic tests to evaluate respiratory distress include blood gas, CBC, CXR, soft tissue airway films (may demonstrate supraglottic edema/subcutaneous emphysema), CT scan of the neck, and C-spine films in cases of trauma.

E. Treatment:
  1. Cool humidified room air/oxygen helps to prevent crust formation.
  2. Oxygen per nasal cannula, face mask, nonrebreather.
  3. Heliox refers to a 80%:20% helium-oxygen mixture. It relies on decreased density of helium to transport oxygen past the obstructive site.
  4. Systemic corticosteroids may be used to acutely decrease edema from trauma/infectious etiology [dexamethasone (Decadron) or methylprednisolone (Solu-Medrol IV)].
  5. Racemic epinephrine works quickly, acting as a topical decongestant; however, it is short acting and there may be a rebound effect once it dissipates.

F. Clinical pearls:
  1. Nasopharyngeal airway is beneficial for patients emerging from general anesthesia or who have mild head trauma but normal respiratory drive. Nasopharyngeal trumpet can be used to open the airway when relaxation of soft palate/base of the tongue occurs.
  2. Oropharyngeal airway may treat ventilatory obstruction due to a relaxed tongue.
  3. Transoral intubation is the standard of airway control. **Contraindications** include C-spine fractures and laryngeal fractures.
  4. Consultation is advised for possible fiberoptic intubation (in cases of difficult intubations), airway distress refractory to

therapeutic options, exam of supraglottis/glottis (i.e., rule out vocal cord paralysis, neoplasm, foreign body).

Tracheotomy

A. The optimal timing for a tracheotomy is controversial. Evaluation of the patient at 7–10 days of intubation is appropriate to assess for likelihood of extubation. If long-term intubation is probable, then a tracheotomy is justified. In some patients with neuromuscular disorders (i.e., Guillain-Barré syndrome) in which longterm vent support is anticipated, earlier tracheotomy may be done.

B. Types: Shiley and Portex tracheostomy tubes are plastic and may be with or without cuffs. Both may be used initially after the surgical procedure. Typically, tracheostomy tubes are kept undisturbed for 3–5 days to allow formation of a well-healed tract. After this point, the plastic tracheostomy tubes are changed to a metal (Jackson) tracheostomy tube for long-term use or Shiley/ Portex trach tubes (cuffed) if ventilatory support is still needed.

C. ENT will do the first tracheostomy change after 3–5 days to ensure a well-healed tract has formed. Frequent cleaning or changing of the inner cannula is recommended to prevent obstruction by crusting (typically at least tid).

- If the trach tube falls out, first assess whether the patient is breathing adequately through the stoma site.
- If the patient is stable and there is no one experienced in trach management, then call the surgical service for assistance.
- If the patient is not stable, then the trach tube usually can be reinserted *with the aid of the obturator.*
- If respirations are still difficult, then the tube is likely in a false tract. The correct tract may be found with the aid of a Kelly clamp to open the stoma site or by passing the trach tube over a fiberoptic scope, suction catheter, or Foley catheter.
- Transoral intubation is always an option.

Epistaxis Emergency

A. *Call a consult immediately for assistance!*

B. Pertinent history: Airway status, history of trauma, anticoagulant medications, systemic diseases (hereditary hemorrhagic telangiectasia or Osler-Weber-Rendu).

C. Pertinent physical exam: Determine the source of bleeding (anterior versus posterior and right versus left nare). Identification of most anterior sites can be aided by nasal speculum and light source (headlight or mirror).

D. Workup: Check coagulation values including bleeding time and hematocrit. Check blood pressure, and treat hypertension.

E. Diagnosis: Bleeding from the nasopharynx or nares causing respiratory distress and aspiration.

F. Treatment:
 1. Epistaxis tray at bedside: nasal speculum, 4% lidocaine, antibiotic/Vaseline-coated gauze for nasal packing, epistaxis

anterior pack (Merocel), Surgicel, silver nitrate sticks, or Epistat (modified Foley balloon with pack) for posterior bleeding.

2. Application of topical vasoconstrictive agents [oxymetazoline hydrochloride (Afrin) 0.05%, phenylephrine hydrochloride 0.25%, or 4% cocaine] may slow down the bleeding.

Epistaxis Urgency

A. Call the ENT resident for an urgent consult.

B. Pertinent history: See previous section regarding pertinent history. Consider local factors including trauma, nasal sprays (decongestants and steroid nasal sprays), foreign bodies, anatomic deformities (septal perforations), nasal prong oxygen, local inflammation due to chronic sinusitis, allergic rhinitis, nutritional deficiencies, and alcohol abuse.

C. Diagnosis: Bleeding from the nasopharynx or nares refractory to *constant* nasal compression for 15–30 minutes at the nasal ala.

D. Treatment:
1. Keep patient seated instead of supine because of risk of choking or swallowing blood.
2. May be managed with selective use of silver nitrate stick if it is a well-visualized anterior bleed.
3. May require either Merocel anterior packing or Vaseline-coated gauze packing for 3–5 days.
4. May require Epistat if there is a posterior bleed refractory to anterior packing.

Epistaxis (General)

A. Clinical pearls:
1. Usually simple nasal compression for 15 minutes will stop the bleeding.
2. Control hypertension.
3. Nasal cannula prongs may irritate and dry the septal mucosa. Replace with humidified O_2 and frequent use of Ocean nasal spray.
4. Do not apply silver nitrate to adjoining sides of the septum. This may lead to a septal perforation.
5. All patients with nasal packing require anti-*Staphylococcus* coverage to reduce chances of toxic shock syndrome.
6. The most common hereditary bleeding disorder associated with epistaxis is von Willebrand's disease.

Acute Sinusitis—Emergency

A. *This is an emergency when the infection has extended past the sinuses—call a consultant immediately!*

B. Pertinent history:

Duration of sinusitis symptoms, vision changes, mental status changes, duration of antibiotic therapy.

Predisposing factors such as malnutrition, diabetes mellitus, chemotherapy, long-term corticosteroids, allergic rhinitis, immunodeficiency states, environmental exposures, and placement of NG tube.

C. Pertinent physical exam: Meningeal signs and orbital signs (proptosis, chemosis, impeded extraocular movement, vision loss). These suggest extension of the infection beyond the sinus and necessitate immediate attention by an ENT consultant.

D. Workup: CT scan of sinus, high-resolution CT scan of orbits to rule out subperiosteal or orbital abscess.

E. Diagnosis: Clinically diagnosed sinusitis with evidence of extension to the intracranial area or orbits.

F. Treatment:
   1. IV antibiotics (broad-spectrum).
   2. Copious use of Ocean nasal spray and Afrin to aid in nasal drainage.
   3. IV steroids to help diminish edema around orbits and reduce optic nerve damage.
   4. Surgery (functional endoscopic sinus surgery) is definitive therapy to drain abscess and sinuses.
   5. If optic nerve damage is imminent, then lateral canthotomy with tendon cantholysis should be done to decrease intraocular pressure.

Vertigo

A. Vertigo emergency
   1. *Important vertigo emergencies* include the following:
      a. Wallenberg's syndrome
      b. Lateral pontomedullary syndrome
      c. Cerebellar hemorrhage
      d. Cerebellar infarction
      e. Vertebrobasilar insufficiency
   2. Pertinent history: Sensation and duration of dizziness, associated symptoms (especially neurologic symptoms), nausea, or vomiting.
   3. Pertinent physical exam: Associated neurologic findings (diplopia, dysphasia, drop attacks, vision loss, dysphagia, loss of pain/temperature sensation, loss of motor control), Horner's syndrome, nuchal rigidity, papilledema, bidirectional gaze-fixation nystagmus, failure of gaze suppression nystagmus, spontaneous upbeat or downbeat nystagmus. Nylen-Barany maneuver: Try to produce the vertigo and nystagmus by having a seated patient quickly lie down while turning his or her head to one side.
   4. Workup: CT/MRI or cerebral angiogram (depending on etiology).
   5. Diagnosis: By clinical exam and supporting imaging studies.
   6. Treatment: Depending on etiology, may include surgical decompression, anticoagulation, and/or supportive care.

B. Vertigo (general)
   1. Call otology service for consult to rule out peripheral etiologies. Commonly seen etiologies by the otolaryngologist:
      a. Benign paroxysmal positional vertigo
      b. Ménière's disease
      c. Vestibular neuronitis
      d. Migraine-associated vertigo
   2. Pertinent history: Information from Vertigo Emergency section, exacerbating factors (especially sudden head motion), associated hearing loss, tinnitus, aural fullness, other otologic symptoms, general medical history, medications.
   3. Pertinent physical exam: Nausea and vomiting (these tend to point to peripheral cause), horizontal nystagmus, fixation suppression of nystagmus, Nylen-Bárány maneuver (reproducible nystagmus and vertigo if seated patient turns head to one side while lying down quickly).
   4. Workup: Rule out medical causes including hypotension or hypertension, cardiac arrhythmias, endocrine abnormalities.
   5. Diagnosis: Mainly clinical diagnosis depending on duration, severity of symptoms, and physical exam.
   6. Treatment:
      a. Compazine suppositories (25 mg pr q6h).
      b. Antivert (12.5–25.0 mg PO q8h prn).
      c. Valium (2–10 mg PO q6h prn).
      d. For severe cases, diazepam (5–10 mg IM) or droperidol (2.5 mg IM).
      e. In general, treatment depends on exact etiology (e.g., BPPV treatment involves Epley or particle repositioning maneuver).

■ PSYCHIATRY
Key Points
A. A patient's right to refuse a psychiatric consultation
   1. Psychiatric consultation in and of itself may be stigmatizing.
   2. Patients have the right to refuse consultation, *unless*
      a. There is concern about the patient being a danger to him- or herself or others.
      b. There is concern about the patient's decision-making capacity.
   3. Clinical pearl: The patient should always be told that a psychiatric consultant is coming to see him or her.

Suicidality
A. When to suspect ideation: When the patient appears sad, depressed, or anxious, when there is a significant drug or alcohol history, when there is a history of domestic abuse, when psychosis is present.
B. Before calling the consult, information includes the following:
   1. Key history: Age, gender, previous psychiatric treatment, suicide plan, presence of psychosis and command hallucina-

tions, presence of anxiety, current meds, brief general medical history, and hospital course.

  2. Key physical findings: Presence or absence of agitation, anxiety, overt psychosis.

C. Treatment:
  1. Keep patient safe; get a sitter until directed otherwise by psychiatry.
  2. Do not let a suicidal patient leave without clearance from psychiatry; once medical issues are resolved, the patient may require transfer to psychiatry, possibly against the patient's wishes.

D. Clinical pearls:
  1. Suicidal ideation is a symptom, not a diagnosis; a full psychiatric interview is necessary to determine the cause and direct treatment.
  2. Never be afraid to ask about the presence of suicidality; you will *not* give the patients ideas they didn't already have.

Violent Patients

A. Critical diagnostic question: Is delirium present (i.e., does the patient have a fluctuating level of consciousness with altered mental status)?

B. Before calling the consult, include the following information:
  1. Key history: Age, gender, onset of symptom, level of orientation, presence of psychosis, prior psychiatric treatment, current meds, brief medical history, and hospital course.
  2. Key physical findings: Vital signs, overt psychosis, localized findings on neurologic exam.

C. Workup: Directed at identifying the cause of the delirium; may include lytes, CBC, U/A, LFTs, CSF studies.

D. Treatment:
  1. Protect the patient and staff; sedate the patient with antipsychotics (e.g., haloperidol IM in doses ranging from 0.5 mg in the frail and elderly to 5 mg in the younger and larger); use restraints if necessary.
  2. Identify and treat the cause of the delirium.
  3. Family members can help reorient delirious patients and lessen their violence. Dimly lit, quiet rooms help, as do glasses and hearing aids for those who need them.

E. Clinical pearls:
  1. Common, less obvious causes of delirium are anticholinergic medications, benzodiazepines, undertreated pain, opiates, and steroids. Offending medicines should be tapered or discontinued as much as possible.
  2. Avoid using benzodiazepines for sedation in delirious patients unless the delirium is from alcohol or sedative withdrawal.
  3. Do not put yourself in danger. Remove all possible items in the vicinity that could be used against you (e.g., stethoscope).
  4. Have security with you.
  5. Stand between the patient and an open door.

Competency

A. Definitions
  1. *Competence* is technically a legal term. Only a judge can declare someone incompetent (and appoint a guardian, for example).
  2. *Decision-making capacity* refers to the ability of patients to give informed consent to medical care; psychiatrists can often assist in the assessment of capacity.
B. Competency is an emergency or urgency as the patient typically requires emergent or urgent medical care for which the patient is unable or unwilling to give consent.
C. Before calling the consult, include the following information:
  1. Key historical information: Age, gender, proposed medical care and risks, benefits, and alternatives particular to the patient, medical history, current meds, presence of psychosis or depression, psychiatric history.
  2. Key physical findings: Presence or absence of agitation, anxiety, overt psychosis.
D. Demonstration of decision-making capacity requires all three of the following:
  1. Understanding of medical situation and likely outcome of no treatment.
  2. Understanding of risks and benefits of treatment options.
  3. Ability to manipulate information rationally and give a rational explanation for preferred treatment.
E. Clinical pearls:
  1. Many consults to psychiatry result from patients not being adequately informed of the proposed treatment's risks and benefits.
  2. Presence of psychosis does not necessarily mean that a patient lacks capacity (e.g., belief that one is part of the intergalactic guard may have no bearing on understanding the risks and benefits of cardiac catheterization).
  3. Capacity is decision specific; one may have capacity to take IV meds but not PO if one believes that all of the pills are sprayed with a poison.
  4. Capacity is time specific. Demonstrating capacity today is no guarantee that one will be able to demonstrate capacity tomorrow should mental status fluctuate.
  5. Psychiatric consultation can only help with determining if a patient lacks capacity to make a decision; the consult will not tell you who the decision-maker should be if the patient lacks capacity.

Psychosis

A. Definition: *Psychosis* is a break with reality demonstrated by hallucinations, delusions, or bizarre behavior.

B. Psychosis itself is not a psychiatric emergency. The psychiatric consult can wait until the morning. On a medical/surgical floor, psychosis is often a symptom of delirium, which can be a medical emergency.

C. Critical diagnostic question: Is the patient delirious (i.e., does the patient have a fluctuating level of consciousness with altered mental status)? If so, see the section on the violent patient for further discussion of delirium.

D. Before calling the consult, include the following information:
   1. Key history: Age, gender, previous psychiatric treatment, nature of psychosis and symptom onset, presence of anxiety, current meds, brief general medical history and hospital course, presence of suicidal or homicidal ideas, presence of command hallucinations.
   2. Key physical findings: Presence or absence of agitation, anxiety, thought disorder, bizarre behavior.

E. Clinical pearls:
   1. Visual hallucinations usually result from delirium or intoxication.
   2. Auditory hallucinations are the most common form in psychiatric disorders.
   3. Olfactory and gustatory hallucinations are usually seen in the aura of a seizure.
   4. Tactile hallucinations can result from drug withdrawal.
   5. Psychosis is a symptom, not a diagnosis; a full psychiatric interview is necessary to determine the cause and direct treatment.

Domestic Violence, Rape, and Psychiatric Trauma

A. Legal reporting requirements:
   1. Physicians in every state are **required** to break confidentiality and report *suspected* cases of child abuse to local authorities, usually called the Division of Family Services or Child Protective Services.
   2. Many states also require that suspected elder abuse be reported.
   3. There are no such legal requirements for spouse abuse.

B. Rape victims should be referred to obstetrics and gynecology for collection of evidence, treatment of physical trauma, possible exposure to STDs, and referred for follow-up counseling.

C. Psychiatric consultation may help with the treatment of depression, anxiety, substance abuse, posttraumatic stress disorder, and personality disorders that are all commonly found in the victims of domestic violence and rape. Perpetrators of domestic violence also frequently have many of these problems.

D. Before calling the consult, make sure the patient is willing to see a psychiatrist. Include the following information:
   1. Key history: Age, gender, previous psychiatric treatment, nature of symptoms, presence of anxiety and depression,

current meds, brief general medical history and hospital course, presence of suicidal or homicidal ideas.
  2. Key physical findings: Presence or absence of agitation, anxiety, overt psychosis.
E. Diagnosis: Questions regarding domestic abuse should be asked as a routine part of the social history on every patient.
F. Treatment:
  1. Should begin with referral to a specific domestic violence support program if one is available locally.
  2. Will depend on the patient's individual symptoms.
  3. Generally includes allowing the patient to tell and retell the story of the trauma in a safe, supportive environment so that the associated anxiety lessens over time.
G. Clinical pearls:
  1. If in doubt about whether to call protective services regarding child abuse for more guidance.
  2. Patients rarely volunteer information on being a victim of domestic violence; the first step toward helping them is to ask.

Chemical Dependency

A. Minor alcohol withdrawal
  1. Diagnosis:
    a. Tremors, headache, nausea, sweating, and autonomic instability occurring approximately 12 hours after the last drink and lasting up to 5 days if untreated.
    b. No hallucinations, seizures, or delirium.
  2. Treatment:
    a. Benzodiazepines given scheduled and prn to keep vital signs stable, with a gradual taper over approximately 4 days.
    b. Frequent monitoring of vital signs.
    c. Adequate hydration.
    d. Adequate replacement of electrolytes, particularly potassium and magnesium, as needed.
    e. Replacement of vitamins, especially vitamin C, folate, and thiamine.
    f. Seizure prophylaxis in those with a history of seizure.
    g. The patient should be encouraged to allow psychiatric consultation for diagnosis and treatment of a possible chemical dependency.
B. Major alcohol withdrawal (a.k.a. *rum fits* and DTs)
  1. This should not result in a straight psychiatric consultation. Consultation with a med-psych service or internal medicine may be appropriate, and such consultation may be emergent.
  2. Diagnosis
    a. See the criteria under minor alcohol withdrawal.
    b. Between 3 days and 2 weeks after the last drink, minor withdrawal symptoms become accompanied by hallucinations, seizures, or delirium. Autonomic instability worsens.

    3. Treatment:
       a. Same as for minor alcohol withdrawal, but monitoring of vital signs and supportive treatment are even more important; severe cases may require transfer to the ICU.
       b. Haloperidol added to the benzodiazepine can help treat hallucinosis.
       c. The patient should be encouraged to allow psychiatric consultation for diagnosis and treatment of a possible chemical dependency.

C. Cocaine and opioid withdrawal
    1. Diagnosis:
       a. In opioid withdrawal: Nausea, muscle aches, rhinorrhea, diarrhea, piloerection, craving.
       b. In cocaine withdrawal: Fatigue, agitation, increased appetite.
    2. Treatment:
       a. While both conditions are unpleasant for the patient, they are rarely medically serious.
       b. Opioid withdrawal can be treated with clonidine, 0.1 mg PO tid or a methadone taper.
       c. The patient should be encouraged to allow psychiatric consultation for diagnosis and treatment of a possible chemical dependency.

D. Chemical dependency
    1. Before calling the consult, make sure the patient is willing to see a psychiatrist. Include the following information:
       a. Key history: Age, gender, previous psychiatric treatment, amount of use, route of use, withdrawal symptoms, presence of anxiety and depression, current meds, brief general medical history and hospital course, presence of suicidal or homicidal ideas, presence of psychosis.
       b. Key physical findings: Presence or absence of agitation, anxiety, overt psychosis, withdrawal signs.
    2. Diagnosis: Questions regarding alcohol and substance use should be asked as a routine part of the social history on every patient.
       a. Criteria revolve around tolerance, withdrawal, and inability to control use.
       b. If two of the CAGE questions (listed here) are positive, the patient should be encouraged to allow psychiatric consultation for more definitive diagnosis. Other patients, of course, may also be appropriate for referral.
          i. Ever tried to *C*ut down
          ii. Had others get *A*nnoyed
          iii. Felt *G*uilty about drinking
          iv. Had an *E*ye opener (morning drink) to avoid withdrawal

3. Treatment:
   a. Support groups such as AA
   b. Anticraving medication such as naltrexone, nalmefene, or ondansetron for alcoholism
   c. Methadone maintenance (from specially licensed clinics) for severe opioid dependence
   d. Psychotherapy aimed at relapse prevention
   e. Treatment of comorbid depression and anxiety disorders
4. Clinical pearls:
   a. Sedative withdrawal has the same clinical picture as alcohol withdrawal.
   b. The shorter the half-life of the benzodiazepine (e.g., alprazolam), the more likely withdrawal.
   c. Untreated DTs has a mortality of over 15%.
   d. Drug use often accompanies STDs, physical trauma, and other medical conditions.

■ GENERAL SURGERY

Key Points

1. Time-efficient communication is crucial. If the surgeon is abrupt, do not take personal offense.
2. Identify yourself and the patient that needs a consult, then clearly identify the question you need answered (i.e., "this is a patient with a pulseless and painful leg").
3. Give an indication of the urgency of the consult (i.e., stat, a few hours, or sometime today).
4. Identify which surgical attending is requested, and then present the crucial information for the problem.
5. If important radiographs have been obtained, state their location (i.e., do not keep them in your callroom).

Hernia

A. *A strangulated hernia is a surgical emergency—call a consult immediately!*
   An incarcerated hernia is not necessarily a surgical emergency. If the hernia is reducible, this is not an urgent consult.
B. Pertinent information: Location and duration of the hernia, scar overlying hernia, associated symptoms, and status (strangulated, incarcerated, or reducible), time of patient's last bowel movement, fever, leukocytosis, or erythema of the skin overlying the hernia. Is the patient immunocompromised?
C. Physical exam: Diagnosis of a hernia is made by examining the patient in a standing position with the patient performing Valsalva's maneuver or coughing. A mass that protrudes is a hernia until proven otherwise. A *reducible* hernia is one that can return through its fascial defect. An *incarcerated* hernia is one that is irreducible

(impossible to push back through the fascial defect). A *strangulated* hernia is one in which the blood flow of the hernia's contents is compromised leading to necrosis of the contained structures. The signs of this are a fever, leukocytosis, hypotension, erythema of the overlying skin, or extreme pain with light palpation of the hernia.

D. Treatment:
   1. Attempt to reduce an incarcerated nonstrangulated hernia that does not protrude inferior to the inguinal ligament.
   2. Place the patient supine in Trendelenburg's position and slowly apply firm, constant, circular pressure with the palm of the hand to the hernia.
      a. If the hernia reduces, then perform an abdominal examination an hour later to prove that ischemic bowel was not reduced. Then, call a non-urgent consult.
      b. If the patient has pain, then call surgery.
   3. Most hernias require an operation if the patient can tolerate the risks of anesthesia.
   4. Trusses or binders are usually not effective in the treatment of hernias.

E. Clinical pearls: Hernias are classified both by anatomy and status. Over 75% of hernias occur in the inguinal region, 10% are incisional or ventral hernias, 3% are femoral, and the remainder are of unusual types. The location is of less concern than the status of the hernia. Not all incarcerated hernias are strangulating. A freely reducible hernia is an elective consult that generally can wait to be requested until the morning.

Ischemic Lower Extremity

A. *Ischemic extremity is an emergency—call a consult immediately!*
B. An ischemic extremity may be due to acute events (embolic disease) or chronic disease (atherosclerosis). The acute event is an emergency because perfusion must be reestablished within 6–8 hours. Unlike patients with chronic disease, these patients have not developed collateral circulation to supply the lower leg.
C. Pertinent information:
   1. Suspected source: Embolism (atrial fibrillation/arrhythmia, LV aneurysm, AAA, or popliteal aneurysm), or chronic disease (atherosclerosis).
   2. Status of the vascular system: Has this patient had vascular surgery, (if so, where does the bypass start and end?), where are the scars, and who was his or her surgeon?
D. Physical exam:
   1. Status of collateral flow: Palpable or Dopplerable pulses in the femoral, popliteal, dorsalis pedis, and posterior tibial arteries. Be able to tell the consultant if there is a temperature difference in the extremities and at what level (foot, shin, thigh, or whole leg).

2. Severity of ischemia: The most sensitive test to determine if the foot is viable is to test for proprioception of the toes. This will diminish within 5 minutes of cessation of blood flow. Next, test motor function and light touch.

E. Treatment options:
   1. Most patients are started on intravenous heparin therapy
   2. Possible interventions include surgical bypass, surgical or interventional radiographic thrombectomy, or locally delivered intravascular thrombolytics.

Ischemic Ulcer of the Lower Extremity

A. Ischemic ulcer of the lower extremity is an elective consult.
B. Pertinent information:
   1. These ulcers are commonly found on the first metatarsal head or tips of the toes and are due to a combination of unrecognized trauma, poor circulation, and infection. These are distinguished from venous stasis ulcers by location (on the lower anterior shin), vascularity (heaped up, engorged edges), and sensitivity (very painful).
   2. Status of the vascular system: Has this patient had vascular surgery (if so, where does the bypass start and end?), and/or where are the scars?
   3. Have any ankle-arm indices been performed (you can call the Vascular Laboratory and they will check the records)?
   4. Are there any radiographs that document osteomyelitis of the underlying bone? Any exposed bone is assumed to have osteomyelitis until proven otherwise.
C. Pertinent physical exam: Palpable or Dopplerable pulses in the femoral, popliteal, dorsalis pedis, and posterior tibial arteries. Signs of infection (e.g., pus discharge with palpation).
D. Treatment options:
   1. Amputation, debridement, or any procedure to increase vascular inflow in arterial disease and promote wound healing
   2. Leg elevation, Unna boots, or compression stockings to encourage venous drainage in venous disease.

Retroperitoneal Bleeding

A. Retroperitoneal bleeding is an urgent consult.
   Retroperitoneal bleeding is most commonly seen in patients after coronary angiography and is partially due to the frequent use of anticoagulant and antiplatelet medications. The hallmark for diagnosis is a decreasing hematocrit in a patient complaining of flank, back, or abdominal pain.
B. Pertinent information: What procedure was performed? What anticoagulants and antiplatelet agents were used, and have they been stopped? How much and over what time period has the hematocrit decreased? On the CT scan (go see it yourself; do not trust the radi-

ologist), how large is it (in centimeters)? Does it compress the urinary system causing hydronephrosis or hydroureter, or compress the renal vein? These last two findings may necessitate urgent percutaneous nephrostomy tubes or surgery, respectively.

C. Pertinent physical exam: Neurologic status of the patient's ipsilateral leg? Test this by asking the patient to straight leg lift and then test light touch on the medial and lateral upper thigh. If these senses are diminished, the patient may need urgent operative decompression of the hematoma.

D. Diagnosis: Abdominal CT scan secures the diagnosis.

E. Treatment options:
   1. Variable treatment depending on situation.
   2. Check CBC immediately and frequently thereafter.
   3. Reverse anticoagulation (Vitamin K, FFP).
   4. Supportive measures (fluids, blood) and/or operative intervention.

Femoral Artery Pseudoaneurysm

A. *Emergency consult if there is compression of the femoral nerve;* it is urgent in most other cases.

B. Pertinent information: This complication of arterial puncture occurs in the same patient population as retroperitoneal hemorrhages. What procedure was performed? What anticoagulants and antiplatelet agents were used, and have they been stopped? How large is the pseudoaneurysm by ultrasound and does it have a long, thin neck? These pseudoaneurysms are more likely to spontaneously thrombose or be amenable to ultrasound-guided compression.

C. Physical exam: The hallmark of diagnosis is a thrill or bruit over the puncture site. Is there any evidence of emboli to the ipsilateral foot. Look at the tips of the toes and search for petechiae or new larger purple or black spots. If present, the patient may need immediate operative intervention. Is there any evidence of compression of the femoral nerve? Test motor function and light touch sensation in the leg. If absent, the patient may need immediate operative intervention.

D. Diagnosis: Ultrasound secures the diagnosis.

E. Treatment options: Vary from expectant management to ultrasonic compression or operative closure of the arteriotomy and evacuation of the hematoma.

Small Bowel Obstruction

A. Small bowel obstruction is an urgent consult. The most common causes are hernias, previous abdominal operations, and carcinoma.

B. Pertinent information: The hallmarks of diagnosis are abdominal distension, nausea, vomiting, waves of abdominal pain progressing to constant pain (an ominous sign), and cessation of bowel movements. Which symptoms are present? How long have they been present? When was the patient's last bowel movement?
Is the patient febrile (and do they have a leukocytosis)?

Are there any hernias?

Have they had any previous abdominal or pelvic operations?

What is the NG tube and Foley catheter output?

C. Physical exam: Check for hernias in the groin, umbilicus, and all scars for incisional hernias.

D. Diagnosis: What does the obstructive series show (do not order a KUB), and is there colonic or rectal air? Most important, does the radiograph demonstrate any free air?

E. Treatment options:
1. Most patients without hernias who have not had previous abdominal operations will need to go to the operating room fairly soon.
2. In those that have had a previous abdominal operation:
   a. Make patient NPO.
   b. Nasogastric decompression.
   c. Fluid resuscitation.
   d. Frequent abdominal exams.
   e. Call surgery immediately if symptoms worsen.

F. Clinical pearls: Most common causes of SBO are hernias, previous abdominal operations, and carcinomas.

Hints for Diagnosis of an Acute Abdomen

An acute abdomen is an abdominal examination that warrants immediate surgical intervention. These hints are not rigid rules because the diagnosis of an acute abdomen can require much judgment. The most common signs indicating an acute abdomen are peritoneal signs due to peritoneal inflammation.

. . . If there is any doubt at all, call. . . .

Signs:

- Rebound: This should never be tested for by pushing into the patient's abdomen and releasing. Not only is it barbaric but also not sensitive. Instead, pain with percussion on the anterior abdominal wall is the best test.
- Tussion: A patient who can cough several times probably does not have peritoneal signs.
- Laughing: A patient who laughs probably does not have peritoneal signs.
- Sitting up for posterior chest auscultation or rolling over for a rectal examination: Most patients with peritoneal signs will not do this.

Abdominal Pain and a Pulsatile Abdominal Mass

A. *Abdominal pain and a pulsatile abdominal mass are an incredible emergency!*

B. Abdominal pain and a pulsatile abdominal mass are the easiest problems you will ever evaluate:
1. Call surgery for a stat consult.
2. Type and cross the patient for six units of blood.

Pneumothorax

A. Pneumothorax is an urgent consult. **Stat** consult if the patient is receiving positive pressure ventilation.

The most common cause of a pneumothorax is a misplaced central venous cannula.

Get a chest tube tray and 22 French chest tube to the bedside.

B. Pertinent information:

Which side?

Where is the CXR?

Is the patient on positive pressure ventilation? If so, this can be very dangerous and you must carefully monitor the patient until tube thoracostomy is performed. If the patient decompensates, place a 14 or 16 angiocatheter in the second interspace at the mid-clavicular line of the affected side.

C. Treatment: Options vary as to the size and the physiologic impact of the pneumothorax:

1. Expectant management with serial chest radiographs may suffice in a young patient with negative pressure ventilation and no shortness of breath.

2. Needle aspiration of the air collection may be chosen.

3. Other patients may require open tube thoracostomy or percutaneous tube thoracostomy (a 14 French Thal tube).

Perirectal Abscess

A. Generally this is an urgent consult unless the patient is **septic**, then it is stat! Remember that there is no such thing as an unimportant abscess. It should always be evaluated by a surgeon.

B. Pertinent information: Is the patient diabetic or immunosuppressed? If so then they are far more likely to die or have greater morbidity from this disease.

Is the patient febrile and do they have a leukocytosis?

C. Physical exam:
- Where is it (relative to the scrotum/vagina, and anus)?
- How far does the erythema and induration extend? If the stigmata of infection extends out from the anus, then the patient may have a Fournier's gangrene, which is a surgical emergency.

D. Treatment options:

1. Incision and drainage either at the bedside or in the operating room.

2. Fournier's gangrene will necessitate wide debridement in the operating room with massive irrigation of affected areas.

3. IV antibiotics.

E. Clinical pearls: "Perirectal abscess" is a misnomer. According to Park's classification system, there is no such thing as a perirectal abscess.

18

Guide to Procedures

. . . It's just a little sting, you won't feel a thing . . .

TABLE 18-1. ALL YOU REALLY NEED TO KNOW ABOUT VASCULAR ACCESS

Type	Description	Common Uses	Duration of Use
Triple-lumen catheter	• 3 separate lumens • Placed via the Seldinger technique usually at the bedside • Subclavian or internal jugular veins preferred, femoral vein can be used	• When peripheral access is exhausted and in emergency situations • Blood may be drawn from the catheter	• Short-term use (~7 days) • Replace femoral lines more frequently (~3 days)
Hickman catheter	• Surgically placed (single or multi-lumen) • Subcutaneously tunneled • Dacron cuff at the skin entry site • Located in subclavian vein (tip is located near the right atrium)	• Long-term intravenous medications and/or fluids • Blood may be drawn from the catheter	• Long-term use • May be left in place indefinitely as long as functioning properly
Hohn catheter	• Single- or double-lumen Silastic catheters • Placed via Seldinger technique by interventional radiology or surgery **without** a subcutaneous tunnel • Antimicrobial cuff at the skin insertion site • Located in subclavian or internal jugular veins	• Placed when peripheral access is exhausted • Administration of medications and fluids (when double-lumen) • Blood may be drawn from the catheter	• Intermediate-term use (up to 6 weeks)

(continued)

TABLE 18-1. ALL YOU REALLY NEED TO KNOW ABOUT VASCULAR ACCESS (Continued)

Type	Description	Common Uses	Duration of Use
Implanted venous access device (Port-A-Cath)	• Placed subcutaneously by a surgeon or interventional radiology • Single or double lumen • Specialized right-angle needle is required to access the portal chamber • Located in subclavian vein; tip is located near the right atrium	• Long-term intravenous medications and/or fluids • Blood may be drawn from the catheter	• Intended for indefinite use
Midline catheter	• *Kink proof* material • Peripherally placed by trained nursing personnel • Located in antecubital vein • Consider the possibility of midline catheter placement early before potential peripheral vessels are damaged	• Intermediate-term intravenous medications are planned (e.g., a several week course of antibiotics) • Not intended for TPN or chemotherapy • Blood drawing is discouraged (causes fibrin deposition at the tip and eventual catheter failure)	• Intermediate-term use (1–6 weeks) • Heparin flushing should be performed when the catheter is not being used for therapy at least twice a day
PICC	• 17-inch Silastic catheter placed by trained nursing personnel • Interventional radiology can place PICC lines under fluoroscopy if necessary • Located in basilic, cephalic, or median cubital vein	• Long-term intravenous medications are planned • TPN and more irritating medications provided the tip is in the superior vena cava • Blood may be drawn from the catheter	• Long-term use • May be left in place indefinitely as long as functioning properly

Complications may include bleeding, pneumothorax, infection, and thrombosis. Clotted catheters may be opened with urokinase.

VENIPUNCTURE

Indications:

- Obtain venous blood for laboratory testing.

Contraindications:

- Cellulitis, phlebitis, or venous obstruction at the site of veni-puncture
- Lymphangitis of the arm
- Venipuncture site proximal to a peripheral IV site

What to Tell the Patient:

A sample of blood will be taken from a vein. There may be a minor amount of pain. Bruising does sometimes occur after venipuncture. Informed consent is not required.

Equipment:

- Tourniquet.
- Gloves.
- Alcohol prep swab.
- Vacutainer hub and appropriate needle. A 20-gauge needle and an appropriate sized syringe may also be used.
- Needles smaller than 22-gauge should be avoided because of the increased risk of hemolysis.
- Appropriate specimen tubes, labeled.
- Gauze pad and bandage.
- Patient labels.

Procedure:

1. Apply the tourniquet above the antecubital fossa. Be careful that it is not so tight as to be uncomfortable.
2. Select an appropriate vein for venipuncture (usually the most easily palpable).
3. Swab the area with the alcohol prep pad.
4. Apply traction to the skin below the proposed site with the non-dominant hand.
5. Holding the syringe or vacutainer in the dominant hand, enter the skin at a 15- to 30-degree angle with the needle bevel up either directly above or along side the vein. Then carefully advance the needle into the vein.
6. Either apply gentle back pressure on the syringe or press the first collection tube onto the needle inside the vacutainer hub.
7. Collect the quantity of blood required and/or fill and mix all the collection tubes.
8. Remove the tourniquet, withdraw the needle, and apply pressure to the site.

9. Apply the bandage.
10. Dispose of the needle properly.

Complications:

- Hematoma
- Phlebitis

FEMORAL VEIN PHLEBOTOMY

Indications:

- Femoral vein phlebotomy may be performed when it is impossible or impractical (e.g., emergency situations) to obtain blood from the arm.

Contraindications:

- Cellulitis or venous obstruction at the site of venipuncture
- Femoral vascular prosthesis over the site of venipuncture
- Anticoagulation or bleeding disorder (relative contraindication)

What to Tell the Patient:

A sample of blood will be taken from a vein in the groin. There will be more pain than from a typical venipuncture. Hematoma formation is not uncommon. The patient should lie supine with the ipsilateral thigh slightly abducted and externally rotated. Informed consent is not required.

Equipment:

- Gloves.
- Alcohol prep swabs.
- An 18- or 20-gauge 1½-inch needle and an appropriate sized syringe may also be used. A vacutainer hub and needle may also be used.
- Appropriate specimen tubes, labeled.
- Gauze pad and bandage.
- Patient labels.

Anatomy:

The structures of the groin lie in the following order from lateral to medial: femoral nerve, femoral artery, femoral vein, empty space, and lymphatics (**NAVEL**). The femoral vein is directly medial to the femoral artery. The femoral pulse is easily palpated in most patients (Fig. 18-1).

Procedure:

1. Determine the approximate location of the femoral vein by palpating the femoral pulse below the inguinal ligament.
2. Cleanse the area.

FIGURE 18-1. The structures of the groin.

3. Place the index and middle fingers of the nondominant hand over the femoral pulse (be careful not to contaminate the area just cleaned).
4. Holding the syringe or vacutainer in the dominant hand, insert the needle perpendicular to the skin just medial to the femoral artery.
5. Advance the needle slowly and smoothly while applying gentle back pressure. If there is no blood return and the needle is inserted to the hub, slowly withdraw the needle while continuing to apply gentle

back pressure. If there is still no blood return, redirect the needle a bit more medially. If there is bright red blood return, the femoral artery has probably been entered. Go ahead and draw the blood that is required. Pressure will need to be applied for a longer duration.

6. Withdraw the appropriate amount of blood (or fill all specimen tubes).
7. Remove the needle and apply direct pressure with gauze for approximately 5 minutes.
8. Fill and mix the specimen tubes. An assistant is helpful at this point so that the phlebotomist can continue to hold pressure. In patients with a bleeding disorder, longer direct pressure is necessary.
9. Apply the bandage.
10. Dispose of the needle properly.

Complications:

- Arterial puncture
- Hematoma
- Arteriovenous fistula (possible following repeated femoral phlebotomies on the same side)

PERIPHERAL IV

From time to time the house staff will be called on to place peripheral IVs. When you are asked, generally the nurse and IV therapist have been unsuccessful. Therefore, the IVs that you place will usually be fairly challenging.

Indications:

- To gain peripheral intravenous access for the administration of fluids, medications, and/or blood.

Contraindications:

- Cellulitis at the proposed site
- Phlebitis or edema of the arm
- Prior ipsilateral mastectomy or other axillary surgery in which venous drainage may be impaired

What to Tell the Patient:

A small plastic catheter is going to be inserted into a vein in the hand or arm in order to give fluids and medications. There will be some minor pain with insertion. Patient cooperation is particularly important. Informed consent is not required.

Equipment:

- Tourniquet.
- Gloves.
- Alcohol prep swabs.
- Povidone iodine prep swabs.

- IV fluids.
- IV tubing.
- Appropriate catheter. A large gauge catheter must be used for infusion of viscous solutions such as blood and blood components (20-gauge or larger). For standard IV solutions and short-term infusions, a smaller catheter is acceptable (22-gauge). The smaller the catheter, the less the irritation to the vein.
- Occlusive dressing and tape.

Anatomy:

Potential areas of insertion include the forearm, the dorsum of the hand, and the antecubital fossa. The most common sites are the veins of the hand, wrist, and forearm. The antecubital fossa should be avoided as bending of the elbow will disturb, occlude, and possibly dislodge the catheter. Always start at the most distal point of the extremity (e.g., the hand) if veins are present. Save the forearm and upper arm for later sites if possible. The lower extremities should *never* be used for IV placement.

Procedure:

1. Assemble the fluids and tubing. Run fluid through the line, flushing all air, and recap the tubing.
2. Apply the tourniquet 4–6 inches above the proposed insertion site. Venous blood flow may also be occluded with a blood pressure cuff, but it should not obstruct arterial flow.
3. Select the vein to be used. Palpation is more important than visualization. Be sure the segment is long enough for the entire catheter.
4. Using a vigorous circular motion, prep the skin with alcohol. Allow to dry.
5. Using a circular motion, work from the center of the insertion site outward with the povidone iodine swab. Allow to dry.
6. Hold the skin taut and anchor the vein with the thumb of the non-dominant hand. Avoid recontamination of the insertion site.
7. Holding the catheter/needle assembly in the dominant hand, lower the hub of the needle close to the skin and align needle for insertion.
8. Insert the needle, bevel up, into the skin and subsequently into the vein. The skin may be punctured at the side of the vein or directly over it. In the side entry technique, the needle should puncture the skin on one side of the vein approximately $1/2$–1 inch below where the needle will enter the vein. Pierce the skin at a 45-degree angle along the side of the vein. Once through the skin, reduce the angle to approximately 20 degrees and enter the vein nearly parallel to the vessel. In the other technique, the skin should be punctured at a 45-degree angle directly over the vein. The angle is reduced to approximately 20 degrees and the vein is entered. If the needle is in the vein, blood return will be visible in the flashback chamber. Advance the needle a few more millimeters.

9. Release the tourniquet.
10. Carefully withdraw the needle approximately ½ inch while continuing to advance the catheter. Apply pressure to the vein just above the tip of the catheter to obstruct blood flow. Remove the needle. *Never* reinsert the needle or pull the catheter back over the needle as this can shear off the plastic tip.
11. Connect the IV tubing to the catheter. To be certain the catheter is in the vein, lower the infusion bag below the level of the insertion site. Blood should appear in the tubing.
12. Cover the insertion site with a transparent occlusive dressing and tape securely.

Complications:

- Hematoma
- Phlebitis
- Cellulitis
- Sepsis
- Extravasation of fluids and/or medications

BLOOD CULTURES

Indications:

- Documentation of bacteremia

Contraindications:

- Similar to those listed under venipuncture

What to Tell the Patient:

Two separate samples of blood are going to be collected for testing and two different needle sticks will be required. Informed consent is not required.

Equipment:

- Venipuncture supplies (previously listed)
- Sterile gloves
- Alcohol prep swab sticks
- Povidone iodine prep swab sticks
- Blood culture bottles
- Patient labels

Procedure:

1. Apply the tourniquet and select a venipuncture site. Release the tourniquet.
2. Vigorously cleanse the skin with three alcohol swab sticks. Work from the proposed puncture site outwards.
3. Swab the area concentrically with three povidone iodine swab sticks. Allow the skin to air dry.

4. Replace the tourniquet.
5. Do not touch the site unless wearing sterile gloves.
6. Perform the venipuncture and collect 20 cc of blood.
7. Without changing the needle, distribute 10 cc of blood to each of the culture bottles. Changing the needle may serve as a source of contamination. Gently mix the contents of the bottle.
8. Label each specimen bottle. The label should also have the drawer's initials, date and time, the word "blood" and the site (e.g., L arm). The specimen may be rejected if it is not properly labeled. Apply direct pressure with gauze over the puncture site and cover with bandage.
9. In almost all instances, you will obtain a second "set" of blood cultures from another site. If you must obtain the second set from the same site, wait approximately 5 minutes and follow the same disinfecting procedures *again*.

Complications:

- Hematoma
- Phlebitis

ARTERIAL BLOOD GAS SAMPLING

Indications:

- To obtain arterial blood for determination of blood gases

Contraindications:

- No palpable radial pulse (the preferred site, followed by the femoral then the brachial arteries)
- Poor collateral circulation in the hand (positive Allen's test)
- Cellulitis over the radial artery
- Anticoagulation or bleeding disorder (relative contraindication)

What to Tell the Patient:

A sample of blood is going to be obtained for testing from an artery in the wrist. It can be quite painful compared to venipuncture. Patient cooperation is particularly important. Informed consent is not required.

Equipment:

- Gloves.
- Alcohol prep swab.
- ABG kit. If a kit is not available, a 3- to 5-cc syringe with a 23- to 25-gauge needle may also be used. The syringe should be heparinized by drawing up 0.5–1 cc of 1:1,000 heparin. Pull the plunger all the way back and then expel all the heparin.
- Ice in a cup or plastic bag.
- Gauze pad and bandage.
- Patient labels.

Procedure:

1. Palpate the radial artery. Perform an Allen's test. Ask the patient to make a tight fist. Occlude the radial and ulnar arteries at the wrist. Have the patient relax the hand. Release the ulnar artery only. The hand should flush red in 5–6 seconds. If color return is delayed there may be poor collateral flow, and a radial artery puncture should not be done on that side.
2. For femoral artery puncture, palpate the femoral pulse just below the inguinal ligament. Remember the mnemonic "NAVEL" (refer to Fig. 18-1).
3. Carefully palpate the chosen artery to determine where pulsations are the most prominent.
4. Swab the area with the alcohol prep pad.
5. Hold the syringe like a pencil. Point the needle proximally with the bevel up. Enter the skin at a 60- to 90-degree angle. Advance slowly until there is a flash of blood. If no flash is encountered, slowly withdraw the needle and continue to look for the flash.
6. Gently aspirate 1–2 cc of blood. The syringe may fill on its own.
7. Quickly remove the needle and apply firm pressure for 5 minutes.
8. Expel any air from the top of the syringe. Roll the syringe gently to mix so that it does not clot.
9. Dispose of the needle properly and cap the syringe.
10. Label the syringe and put it on ice.
11. Be sure the specimen gets to the lab as soon as possible.

Complications:

- Hematoma
- Infection
- Thrombosis of the radial artery; ischemia of the hand

CENTRAL VENOUS ACCESS

The most common sites for a central line are the right internal jugular vein, the subclavian veins, and the femoral veins. The usual method of obtaining central venous access is the over-the-wire technique (Seldinger's technique). The vein is first entered with a needle. A guidewire is passed through this needle. The needle is then withdrawn. The vessel is dilated. The catheter is then fed into the vein over the wire. **The most crucial part of the procedure is keeping hold of the guidewire. Never, ever let go of it.** *(Do you really want to be forever known as the intern that let go of the wire?)* It will be assumed that triple lumen catheter kits that contain most of the necessary equipment (e.g., catheter, wire, dilator, needles, suture, anesthetic, etc.) are available.

Indications:

- Emergency venous access
- Exhausted peripheral access

- Rapid large volume fluid administration
- TPN administration
- Administration of multiple incompatible intravenous medications

Contraindications:
- Thrombosis of the selected vein
- Unexplained edema of the face and/or associated arm or leg
- Infection or cellulitis over the proposed site
- Previous surgery in the proposed area
- Anticoagulation or bleeding disorder (relative contraindication)

What to Tell the Patient:
A large catheter will be placed in a large vein in order to provide better care. There are risks (see the following). The patient will experience some pain with the procedure. Positioning and cooperation are critical and should be explained to the patient in advance. **Informed consent is required.**

Equipment:
- Sterile gloves
- Appropriate materials to cleanse the skin (if not included in the kit)
- Gown, mask, goggles
- Sterile drapes (if not included in the kit or if you want extra, which is always a good idea)
- Extra syringes, local anesthetic, and saline flush (just in case)
- Small syringes with normal saline to flush the catheter lumens after insertion
- Triple lumen catheter kit

Anatomy:
- The internal jugular vein runs medial to the upper portion of the sternocleidomastoid muscle, deep to the triangle formed by the two heads of the mid-portion of the muscle, and then joints with the subclavian vein. The carotid artery is medial to the internal jugular vein (Fig. 18-2).
- The subclavian vein travels under the clavicle near apex of the lung. The subclavian artery is above and behind the vein (see Fig. 18-4).
- See Fig. 18-1 for the anatomy of the structures in the inguinal region.

Procedure:
Right Internal Jugular Vein (Central Approach)
1. Obtain informed consent.
2. Enlist someone else to be your nonsterile assistant.
3. Place the patient in the Trendelenburg position. Have the patient turn his/her head to the left approximately 45 degrees.
4. Don goggles, mask, gown, and gloves.

5. Cleanse the site.
6. Drape the field.
7. Identify the apex of the triangle formed by the heads of the sterno-cleidomastoid muscle and also the carotid artery (refer to Fig. 18-2 for procedure).
8. Anesthetize the area.
9. Using a 22-gauge 2-inch needle and syringe, bevel up, at about a 30- to 45-degree angle to the plane of the patient, directed to the ipsilateral nipple attempt to locate the vein. Palpate the carotid artery with the nondominant hand as you go. The vein is usually encountered between 2–4 cm but can be more superficial. If unsuccessful, slowly withdraw the needle while aspirating. If there is still no venous blood return, redirect the needle slightly more laterally and then slightly more medially (*keep your fingers on the carotid artery*) while applying back pressure. If still unsuccessful, critically reassess the landmarks and patient positioning (Fig. 18-3).

FIGURE 18-2. Central venous access.

FIGURE 18-3. Accessing the right internal jugular vein (central approach).

10. If the carotid artery is inadvertently entered (bright red pulsatile blood that fills the syringe without back pressure), remove the needle and apply direct pressure for 10–15 minutes.
11. When venous blood is obtained, memorize the site and angle. Withdraw the needle.
12. Reinsert the large introducer needle supplied with the kit into the same site at the same angle until venous blood freely flows into the syringe again.
13. Securely hold the needle and remove the syringe. Always keep a finger over the open end of the needle to help reduce the risk of air embolization.
14. Gently pass the guidewire through the needle. It should advance easily without resistance. If resistance is met, remove the wire and check the needle placement again by replacing the syringe and withdrawing blood. Attempt to reintroduce the guidewire.
15. Leave enough of the guidewire outside the patient to accommodate the length of the catheter.
16. **While holding the guidewire's distal end** remove the introducer needle from the patient. Now **hold the wire where it exits the skin** and slide the needle completely off the wire.

17. Nick the skin with a scalpel to enlarge the puncture site.
18. Thread the dilator onto the guidewire and gently into the vein. Remove the dilator. **Never lose hold of the guidewire.**
19. Thread the catheter onto the guidewire. **Do not pass the catheter into the vein until you have a firm hold on the distal end of the guidewire.** Pass the catheter into the vein **while continuously holding the distal end of the guidewire**. Open the distal port to accommodate distal end of guidewire.
20. While holding the catheter in place remove the guidewire.
21. Confirm placement by withdrawing venous blood from all ports. Flush the ports.
22. Securely suture the catheter in place.
23. Apply povidone iodine ointment and an occlusive dressing.
24. Start IV fluids at a minimal rate.
25. Obtain a stat CXR to confirm the location of the catheter (tip should be in the SVC near the right atrium) and rule out pneumothorax.
26. Write a procedure note, whether or not you were successful.

Subclavian Vein

1. Follow steps 1 and 2 above for right internal jugular placement.
2. Patient positioning is especially important for successful subclavian placement. Place the patient in the Trendelenburg position. Place a towel roll between the scapulae and allow the shoulder to fall backwards. Both arms should be extended at the patient's sides. If the catheter will be inserted on the left (preferred), turn the patient's head to the right. If working on the right, turn the head to the left.
3. Follow previous steps 4, 5, and 6.
4. Place the index finger of the nondominant hand at the sternal notch. Place the thumb of the same hand at the point where the clavicle bends over the first rib (approximately the junction of the lateral one-third and the medial two-thirds of the length of the clavicle). The subclavian vein should traverse a line between the thumb and index finger (Fig. 18-4).
5. With a small gauge needle, anesthetize the skin and subcutaneous tissue just below the clavicle and lateral to the thumb.
6. Enter the skin with the introducer needle with the bevel facing up, lateral to the thumb and just caudal to the clavicle. While aspirating, slowly advance the needle under the clavicle toward the index finger parallel to the floor at all times. You may need to depress the needle with your thumb to get under the clavicle. When the needle enters the vein there should be free return of dark blood. If there is no blood return after 5 cm, slowly withdraw the needle while continuing to aspirate. If there is still no blood return, redirect the needle to slightly above the sternal notch. Multiple attempts to redirect the needle are inadvisable (Fig. 18-5).
7. Once there is good venous return, rotate the syringe and needle so that the bevel is toward the feet.

8. Follow previous steps 14 through 27. If there is resistance to guidewire passage after it has cleared the tip of the needle, it may be going upward into the internal jugular vein. Remove the guidewire. Reconfirm the location of the needle by replacing the syringe and withdrawing venous blood. Turn the patient's head toward you and gently try to pass the guidewire again. Introduce the dilator only approximately 3–4 cm.

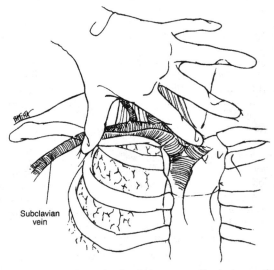

FIGURE 18-4. Subclavian vein should traverse a line between the thumb and index finger.

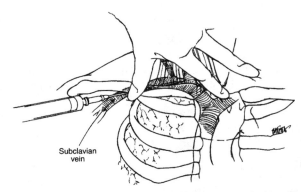

FIGURE 18-5. When the needle enters the subclavian vein there should be free return of dark blood.

Femoral Vein

1. Obtain informed consent and enlist someone else to be your non-sterile assistant.
2. Place the patient in the supine position with the ipsilateral thigh slightly abducted and externally rotated.
3. Follow steps 4, 5, and 6 under Right Internal Jugular Placement.
4. Determine the approximate location of the femoral vein by palpating the femoral pulse below the inguinal ligament, using the "NAVEL" mnemonic (see Fig. 18-1).
5. Anesthetize the area with a small gauge needle. Be sure to aspirate before injecting.
6. While palpating the femoral artery, enter the skin below the inguinal crease and approximately 1 cm medial to the pulse with the introducer needle attached to a syringe at an approximate 30- to 45-degree angle, directed cephalad, and bevel up. While applying back pressure, advance the needle slowly and smoothly until there is free return of venous blood (Fig. 18-6). If there is no return after approximately 5 cm, slowly withdraw the needle while continuing to aspirate. If there is still no return, redirect the needle slightly more lateral. If there is return of arterial blood, withdraw the needle and hold firm pressure for approximately 10–15 minutes.
7. Follow steps 14 through 24 and 27 under Right Internal Jugular Placement once there is good venous return.

FIGURE 18-6. Accessing the femoral vein.

Complications:
- Inadvertent arterial puncture
- Pneumothorax
- Hemothorax/hydrothorax
- Retroperitoneal bleeding
- Cardiac tamponade
- Air embolus
- Hematoma
- Cellulitis
- Line sepsis (most common with femoral lines)
- Thrombosis/embolism

Arterial Line Placement

The preferred site for arterial cannulation is the radial artery. The technique can be difficult even for the experienced operator. The femoral artery is an alternative site.

Indications:
- Continuous arterial pressure monitoring.
- Frequent blood gas monitoring.

Contraindications:
- Poor collateral circulation of the hand (e.g., failed Allen's test)
- Prior vascular bypass surgery, aneurysm, or severe atherosclerosis of the femoral artery
- Anticoagulation or bleeding disorder (relative contraindication)
- Cellulitis over the proposed site

What to Tell the Patient:

A catheter will be placed into an artery in the wrist or the groin in order to monitor blood pressure and/or to obtain frequent arterial blood samples. The procedure can be quite painful. **Informed consent is required.**

Equipment:
- Sterile gloves.
- Appropriate materials to cleanse the skin (if not included in the kit).
- Gown, mask, goggles.
- Sterile drapes.
- Gauze sponges.
- Arm board and tape (radial artery only).
- Pressure infusion bag, pressure tubing, dilute heparin flush, appropriate transducer, and monitor (the ICU nurse will almost always know exactly what this entails and get it set up for you in advance so be sure to let him/her know that you plan to place an arterial line).
- Local anesthetic and small needles and syringes for administration.

- 20-gauge 1½–2-inch Angiocath or quick catheter (radial artery) or 18-gauge introducer needle, guidewire, and 16-gauge, 6-inch arterial catheter (femoral artery).
- Suture.
- Sterile occlusive dressing.

Procedure:

Radial Artery

1. Obtain informed consent.
2. Enlist someone else to be your nonsterile assistant (the ICU nurse is a good idea, as he or she will need to connect the line to the transducer and the transducer to the monitor).
3. Perform the Allen's test on the proposed side. Proceed only if there is good collateral flow.
4. Dorsiflex the patient's wrist and place a towel or gauze roll underneath. Secure the palm and forearm to an arm board with tape.
5. Don goggles, mask, gown, and gloves.
6. Cleanse the site.
7. Drape the field.
8. Carefully palpate the radial artery. Administer local anesthetic to the skin and subcutaneous tissue in this area. Be sure to aspirate before and injecting and do not aim directly for the artery.

FIGURE 18-7. Accessing the radial artery.

9. Puncture the skin at a 45-degree angle with the 20-gauge Angiocath, pointing proximal, bevel up. Slowly and smoothly advance the catheter and needle (Fig. 18-7). When the artery is punctured there will be a flash of bright red blood into the hub. If there is no

flash, withdraw slowly and continue to watch for the flash. If there is still no flash, redirect toward the point of maximal pulsation again and advance carefully at a slightly steeper angle.

10. Once the Angiocath is in the arterial lumen, reduce the angle to approximately 20–30 degrees and advance the needle and catheter slightly (1–2 mm). Carefully slide the catheter off the needle into the lumen. If you are using a quick catheter, advance the guidewire into the artery and then pass the catheter over it. The catheter should pass without resistance. Remove the needle. Either occlude the artery proximally or be ready to put your finger over the catheter opening to prevent the forcible flow of arterial blood.

11. Immediately connect to the pressure tubing. There should be an arterial waveform on the monitor.

12. Suture the catheter in place.

13. Apply the dressing.

14. Write a procedure note, whether or not you were successful.

Femoral Artery

1. Follow steps 1 and 2 above for radial artery cannulation.

2. Place the patient in the supine position with the ipsilateral leg slightly abducted and externally rotated.

3. Locate the point of maximal femoral artery pulsation below the inguinal ligament using the "NAVEL" mnemonic (see Fig. 18-1).

4. Follow previous steps 5, 6, and 7.

5. Anesthetize the skin and subcutaneous tissue over the femoral artery (aspirate before injecting).

6. Using the 18-gauge introducer needle bevel up, puncture the skin at a 45-degree angle over the femoral pulsations. Advance the needle cephalad while continually aspirating. When the femoral artery is entered there should be rapid return of pulsatile bright red blood. If there is no arterial blood after 5 cm, slowly withdraw the needle while aspirating. If there is still no blood return, redirect the needle toward the maximal pulsations and advance again.

7. When the artery is entered, remove the syringe from the introducer needle (be careful to occlude the pulsatile flow of blood with your finger).

8. Advance the guidewire into the artery. It should pass without resistance.

9. **While holding the guidewire's distal end**, remove the introducer needle from the patient. Now **hold the wire where it exits the skin** and slide the needle completely off the wire.

10. Make a small nick in the skin with a scalpel where the wire exits.

11. Thread the catheter onto the guidewire. **Do not pass the catheter into the artery until you have a firm hold on the distal end of the guidewire.** Pass the catheter into the artery **while continuously holding the distal end of the guidewire.**

12. Remove the guidewire and quickly place a finger over the open end of the catheter.
13. Follow previous steps 11 through 14.

Complications:

- Thrombosis of the artery
- Embolization of air, clot, or atherosclerotic material
- Hematoma/hemorrhage
- Retroperitoneal bleeding
- Arteriovenous fistula formation
- Pseudoaneurysm formation
- Ischemia of the supplied area
- Cellulitis, thrombophlebitis, sepsis

LUMBAR PUNCTURE

Indications:

- Analysis of CSF for diagnostic purposes
- Injection of various agents into the CSF (e.g., contrast agent, antibiotics, chemotherapeutic agents)
- Drainage of CSF

Contraindications:

- Known or suspected intracranial mass and/or increased pressure
- Infection over the site
- Anticoagulation, bleeding disorder, or platelets <50K

What to Tell the Patient:

"Spinal taps" are associated with many myths. The procedure is associated with less pain and much less risk than the patient probably imagines. Proper positioning is critical, and you should enlist the patient's assistance with this. **Informed consent is required.**

Anatomy:

In adults the spinal cord usually terminates between L1 and L2. When a lumbar puncture is done, the goal is to obtain fluid from the lumbar cistern below this level. The puncture may be done at the L3/L4, L4/L5 (most common), or L5/S1 interspaces. The line connecting the posterior superior iliac crests (the intercristal line) intersects the spine at either the L4 spinous process or the L4/L5 interspace.

Equipment:

- Sterile lumbar puncture kit
- Extra small gauge needles, syringes, and local anesthetic (just in case)
- Appropriate materials to cleanse the skin (if not included in the kit)

- Sterile gloves
- Mask and goggles

Procedure:

1. Obtain informed consent.
2. Enlist someone else to be your nonsterile assistant (not always necessary but nice to have around).
3. Place the patient in the lateral decubitus position with his or her back close to the edge of the bed or table. The patient should bring the knees up to the abdomen and flex the head to the chest as much as possible. The patient may need assistance holding this position (an assistant is very handy for this purpose). The procedure may also be done with the patient sitting and leaning forward. Obesity, osteoarthritis, and prior lumbar spine surgery may make positioning, identification of landmarks, and successful completion of the procedure very difficult.
4. Palpate the area of the intercristal line. Locate and mark the L4/L5 interspace.
5. Put on sterile gloves.
6. Cleanse the area and drape the patient.
7. Anesthetize the skin with a 25-gauge needle. Anesthetize to deeper structures with a 22-gauge needle.
8. Puncture the skin with spinal needle (stylet in place), bevel up (or parallel to the bodies long axis). Carefully advance the needle between the vertebrae, aiming the tip cephalad at approximately 15–30 degrees (towards the navel), parallel to the floor. A "pop" will often be felt when the subarachnoid space is entered. Remove the stylet and observe for the flow of CSF. It may help to rotate the needle slightly. If there is none, replace the stylet (always be sure to do this) and advance a bit further. Remove the stylet again and so forth. If bone is encountered, pull back 1–2 cm and redirect.
9. When CSF flow is established, attach a manometer and stopcock. Measure the opening pressure (normal 70–180 mm). Collect approximately 3–4 cc of CSF in each tube. If cytology or other studies are to be done, more can be collected.
10. Replace the stylet and withdraw the needle.
11. Place a bandage over the site.
12. Write a procedure note, whether or not you were successful.
13. Instruct the patient to remain recumbent for 4–6 hours.
14. **Send the tubes** as follows: (1) Gram's stain, culture, AFB, fungal stain and culture; (2) glucose and protein; (3) CBC with differential; and (4) special studies as indicated. Refer to the Neurology section (Chapter 17, Fig. 17-3) for interpretation of CSF studies.

Complications:

- Spinal headache
- Trauma to the nerve roots
- Herniation

- Bleeding into the subdural or subarachnoid space
- Meningitis

THORACENTESIS

Indications:

- Obtain pleural fluid for diagnostic testing
- Drainage of pleural fluid in patients with large symptomatic effusions

Contraindications:

- Anticoagulation or bleeding disorder (relative)
- Severely impaired respiratory reserve to the degree that a pneumothorax could not be tolerated (relative)

What to Tell the Patient:

A needle will be inserted through the chest wall to obtain pleural fluid for diagnosis and/or relief of symptoms. Pain is usually mild. Holding still is very important to reduce the risk of pneumothorax. **Informed consent is required.**

Anatomy:

At least 250–300 cc of pleural fluid will be evident as blunting of the costophrenic angle on CXR. Pleural fluid may be loculated, and a decubitus film should be done to determine if the effusion is free flowing. The intercostal vein, artery, and nerve travel in a groove along the inferior margin of the rib. Therefore, the entry site should be at the superior aspect of the rib.

Equipment:

- Sterile thoracentesis kit
- Extra small gauge needles, syringes, and local anesthetic (just in case)
- Appropriate materials to cleanse the skin (if not included in the kit)
- Sterile gloves
- Mask and goggles

Procedure:

1. Obtain informed consent.
2. Enlist someone else to be your nonsterile assistant (not always necessary but nice to have around).
3. Have the patient sit on the edge of the bed leaning forward slightly on a bedside table. Percuss the location of the effusion and mark where the procedure will be attempted on the posterolateral chest.
4. Put on sterile gloves.
5. Cleanse the area and drape the patient.
6. Anesthetize the skin with a 25-gauge needle. Anesthetize to deeper structures including the rib periosteum with a 22-gauge needle.

7. Carefully advance the needle **over the superior aspect of the rib**. Continue to advance slowly until pleural fluid is aspirated.
8. Note the depth and trajectory. Remove the needle.
9. Make a small superficial nick in the skin at the needle entry site (to facilitate easy entry of the catheter/needle assembly).
10. Follow the same path with the catheter/needle assembly (attached to a syringe), aspirating all the way. Be sure to step over the rib.
11. When pleural fluid is obtained, slide the catheter into the pleural space and withdraw the needle. Place a finger over the opening of the catheter. **Never advance the needle back into the catheter.**
12. Attach a 30- to 50-cc syringe with a three-way stopcock to the catheter.
13. Attach connecting tubing to the sidearm of the stopcock. This may be connected to vacuum bottles or a collection bag. Pump out or allow the vacuum to suck out up to 1 L of pleural fluid. Do not collect more than 1 L as this increases the risk of re-expansion pulmonary edema.
14. When finished collecting pleural fluid, have the patient hum or Valsalva and remove the catheter.
15. Bandage the site.
16. Write a procedure note, whether or not you were successful.
17. Obtain a CXR to rule out pneumothorax.
18. **Send pleural fluid** for cell count and differential, Gram's stain, routine culture, fungal stain and culture, specific gravity, protein, LDH, and glucose. If pH will be ordered, the sample must be fresh, in a heparinized syringe, on ice, and taken directly to the lab. Other tests may be done depending on the clinical situation. Refer to the following table regarding the interpretation of pleural fluid studies.

TABLE 18-2. PLEURAL FLUID ANALYSIS

Parameter	Transudate*	Exudate**
Specific gravity	<1.016	>1.016
Total protein (TP) (g/dL)	<3.0	>3.0
Effusion TP/serum TP	<0.5	>0.5
LDH (IU)	<200	>200
Effusion LDH/serum LDH	<0.6	>0.6
Cholesterol	<45	>45
Glucose		Decreased in RA, cancer, TB, and empyema
pH	~7.4	<7.3 suggests TB; <7.2 suggests need for chest tube
Cells	<1,000 WBC <10,000 RBC	>1,000 WBC >10,000 RBC

*CHF, cirrhosis, nephrosis.
**Bacterial or viral pneumonia, empyema, pulmonary infarction, TB, RA, SLE, malignancy, pancreatitis.

Complications:

- Pneumothorax
- Hemothorax
- Re-expansion pulmonary edema

PARACENTESIS

There is no single physical finding that is both highly sensitive and specific for the presence of ascites. The most useful physical findings for making the diagnosis of ascites are a fluid wave, shifting dullness, and peripheral edema. The inability to demonstrate bulging flanks, flank dullness, or shifting dullness are most useful for ruling out ascites.

Indications:

- Obtain ascitic fluid for diagnostic tests.
- Decrease respiratory distress and abdominal discomfort caused by ascites.

Contraindications:

- Anticoagulation or bleeding disorder (relative)
- Uncertainty if abdominal distention is actually caused by fluid
- Bowel obstruction or distended bowel
- Massive obesity (relative)

What to Tell the Patient:

A needle will be used to withdraw fluid from the abdomen for diagnosis and/or relief of symptoms. Have the patient empty their bladder before the procedure. **Informed consent is required.**

Equipment:

- Paracentesis kit that contains a catheter/needle assembly, three-way stopcock, collection tubing, etc. A thoracentesis kit with the same equipment will also work fine.
- Extra small gauge needles, syringes, and local anesthetic (just in case).
- Appropriate materials to cleanse the skin (if not included in the kit).
- Sterile gloves.
- Mask and goggles.

Procedure:

1. Obtain informed consent.
2. Enlist someone else to be your nonsterile assistant (not always necessary but nice to have around).
3. Have the patient lie supine with the head of the bed elevated a bit. Percuss the abdomen to help determine the site for needle entry. Possible entry sites include the midline 3–4 cm below the umbilicus or

the right or left lower quadrants midway between the umbilicus and the anterior superior iliac spine (lateral to the rectus abdominus sheath). Avoid old surgical incisions and areas of skin infection.

4. Put on sterile gloves.
5. Cleanse the area and drape the patient.
6. Anesthetize the skin with a 25-gauge needle. Anesthetize the abdominal wall to the peritoneum with a 22-gauge needle. A 20-gauge spinal needle may be used in very obese patients.
7. Advance the catheter/needle assembly (attached to a syringe) through the skin and abdominal wall aspirating along the way, either at an oblique angle or in a "Z-track" fashion (once the skin is penetrated, the catheter/needle is moved 1–2 cm then advanced further). A small pop may be felt as the needle advances through the fascia.
8. When peritoneal fluid is obtained, slide the catheter into the peritoneal cavity and withdraw the needle. **Never advance the needle back into the catheter**.
9. Attach a 30- to 50-cc syringe with a three-way stopcock to the catheter. If the paracentesis is being done for diagnostic purposes, aspirate the necessary quantity of fluid.
10. If the paracentesis is being done for therapeutic purposes, attach connecting tubing to the sidearm of the stopcock. This may be connected to vacuum bottles or a collection bag. Pump out or allow the vacuum to suck out up to 1 L of ascitic fluid. If the flow of fluid stops, gently manipulate the catheter or reposition the patient. More fluid may be removed from patients with cirrhosis and peripheral edema.
11. Remove the catheter when finished collecting peritoneal fluid.
12. Bandage the site.
13. Write a procedure note, whether or not you were successful.
14. Depending on the clinical situation, **samples should be sent for** the following: cell count and differential, total protein, albumin, LDH, glucose, specific gravity, Gram's stain, routine culture, fungal stain and culture, and AFB stain and culture. The highest culture yields occur when blood culture bottles are inoculated at the bedside. Greater than 250 neutrophils per microliter is suggestive of peritonitis. Other tests (e.g., cytology, amylase, and triglycerides) may be done as the clinical situation dictates. Refer to the following table regarding the interpretation of ascitic fluid studies.

Complications:

- Persistent ascitic fluid leakage
- Bowel perforation
- Hemorrhage
- Peritonitis
- Hypotension, oliguria, and shock
- Bladder perforation

TABLE 18-3. ASCITIC FLUID ANALYSIS

Condition	Protein (g/dL)	SAAG* (g/dL)	LDH (IU)	Glu-cose	WBC (#/cc)	RBC (#/cc)	Amylase
Cirrhosis	<2.5	≥1.1	<200	<60	Low	Low	N/A
CHF	<2.5	≥1.1	<200	>60	Low	Low	N/A
Nephrosis	<2.5	<1.1	<200	>60	Low	Low	N/A
Peritoneal cancer	>2.0	<1.1	>200	<60	High	Very high	N/A
Infection	>2.5	<1.1	>200	>60	Very high	Low	N/A
Pancreatitis	>2.5	<1.1	>200	>60	Vari-able	Vari-able	Very high

*Serum ascites albumin gradient (serum albumin-ascitic fluid albumin).

19

Critical Care Notes

. . . Survival of the fittest . . .

KEYS TO INTENSIVE CARE UNIT SURVIVAL

. . . Always come back to the basics: Air goes in and out. Blood goes round and round. Oxygen is good. . . .

- Transfer notes (see Chapter 6) with key details of the patient's past medical history and course are always helpful. The primary physician, receiving physician, and the patient's family members should be notified. Note any details or special situations that need attention and/or follow up.
- Admitting a patient to an intensive care unit can be intimidating, but keep in mind the ABCs (Airway, Breathing, Circulation) and focus on stabilizing the patient.
- Be nice to the nurses, respiratory therapists, and other ancillary staff during your stay. They can often make useful suggestions, catch things you miss, and be immensely helpful to you in critical situations. They can be the difference between an enjoyable or miserable experience.
- Ask (and keep asking) if you have questions or problems. Mistakes from inexperience in critically ill patients can have catastrophic consequences.
- Always treat the patient, not the numbers.
- It's always a good idea to make rounds on patients and follow up on labs several times a day even if things seem stable.
- Two references to have nearby at all times:

   Marino P. *The ICU Book*, 2nd ed. Baltimore: Williams & Wilkins, 1998.

   Kollef M. Critical care. In *Washington Manual of Medical Therapeutics*, 30th ed. Philadelphia: Lippincott Williams & Wilkins, 2001.

VENTILATORS

. . . Breathe in, breathe out . . .

Suggestions for Initial Ventilator Settings

Mode:
- CMV/AC: Guarantees set tidal volume; often best to start with this.
- SIMV + PSV: Choreographed breaths at preselected rate; allows spontaneous breaths.
- PCV: Pressure ventilation; can't guarantee the tidal volume if lung compliance decreases.

   Tidal volume: 10–12 cc/kg versus 5–7 cc/kg in low tidal volume ventilation.

Rate: 10–15 breaths/minute.

FiO_2: 1.0, then titrate down (patients should never be ventilated on 100% O_2 >24 hours unless absolutely necessary).

PEEP: 0–5 cm H_2O (careful with auto-PEEP).

Inspiratory flow: 50–60 L/min. With COPD may want as high as 100 L/min.

I:E ratio: 1:2. This must be set individually with PCV.

Peak and Plateau pressures: Attempt to keep peak P <45 and plateau P <35.

Ventilator Adjustments

- A Po_2 of 60 mm Hg or greater is usually the goal. Oxygenation is most affected by mean air pressure. Adjustments to FiO_2 and PEEP can help increase oxygenation. Remember that the oxygen saturations tell you nothing about the Pco_2.
- CO_2 Is regulated by ventilation. Increasing the respiratory rate or tidal volume blows off more CO_2.

TABLE 19-1. SUGGESTIONS FOR VENTILATOR MANAGEMENT BASED ON Pco_2 AND Po_2*

	Pco_2	Po_2
High	↑ Minute volume	Decrease FiO_2
	↑ Tidal volume	
	↑ Respiratory rate	
Low	↓ Minute volume	PEEP
	↓ Tidal volume	± Increased FiO_2 (in cases of diffusion block, increase FiO_2)
	↓ Respiratory rate	

*Individualize for every patient.

General "Ballpark" Change Guidelines

- Desired Pao_2 >60. Use the simple ratio (e.g., if Pao_2 is 150 on 100% O_2...

$$\frac{150}{60} = \frac{100}{X} \qquad \therefore X = 40\%).$$

The FiO_2 can be reduced to .40 and this should maintain a Pao_2 of 60.
- Desired Pco_2. Another simple formula:

Pco_2 (current rate) = desired Pco_2 (X)

X = New rate to set to obtain the desired Pco_2

Worsening Oxygenation

The knee-jerk impulse is to turn up the FiO_2. Don't panic, approach the problem in a stepwise manner:

- Is there a ventilator problem?
  Is the ET tube in the correct position or has it migrated? Check with the nurse on the marking of the ET tube and the most recent x-ray.
  Is there a cuff leak or kink in the ET tube? Have respiratory therapy check this.
  Recheck the ventilator settings. Have there been inadvertent changes?
  Is there an obstruction in the ET tube (e.g., mucous plug)? Suction now.
- Is it a patient-related problem (e.g., biting, agitation)? Sedation may be needed.
  Always consider pneumothorax. Listen on both sides and consider a CXR.
  Is the underlying problem worsening? Antibiotic coverage, fluid overload—consider diuretics, bronchodilators. Is a PE a possibility?
  Is the patient oversedated? Do you need to rethink the mode of ventilation? Check the PEEP level at end-expiration. Hypoxemia can be from a loss of PEEP.

Weaning Parameters

- The method of weaning is not as relevant as knowing the appropriate time to wean.
- Factors to consider:
  WEANS NOW mnemonic
  Wakefulness
  Electrolytes
  Acid–base status
  Neurologic state
  Secretions
  Nutrition
  Oxygenation: PaO_2 >60 on FIO_2, 0.4, PEEP <5 cm H_2O
  Work of breathing
- No weaning parameters are perfect. However, one formula often used is the Rapid Shallow Breathing Index (RSBI). If the RSBI is <100 after 1 hour of CPAP with PSV 5 and PEEP 5, the patient is often weanable.

$$RSBI = \frac{\text{Respiratory rate}}{\text{Tidal volume (in liters)}}$$

CARDIAC PARAMETERS

. . . Don't go breaking my heart. . . .
- Normal cardiac output
  5 ± 1 L/min
- Normal cardiac index
  $3 ± 0.54$ min/m^2
- Normal filling pressures
  Right atrial pressure   0–8 mm Hg
  Right ventricular pressure   5–30/0–8 mm Hg
  Pulmonary artery pressure   15–30/3–12 mm Hg
  Pulmonary wedge pressure   3–12 mm Hg

SUGGESTIONS FOR PROPHYLAXIS

. . . An ounce of prevention is worth a pound of cure. . . .

- DVT: SC heparin (5,000 U q8–12h), intermittent pneumatic compression boots.
- GI: Sucralfate, 1 g PO bid, Pepcid, 20 mg IV bid, or Prilosec, 20 mg PO qd.
- Decubitus ulcers: Turn patient several times a day, vigilant skin care, egg crate mattress or Kin-Air bed, and adequate nutrition.
- Deconditioning: Physical therapy and nutritional support.
- Aspiration precautions: Elevate head of the bed and frequent suctioning (especially around the cuff of ET tube).
- Seizure or fall precautions: as appropriate.
- Infection: Maintain oral hygiene, keep track of lines (IV, NG tube, feeding tubes) and change per protocol, and target or discontinue antibiotic therapy to avoid resistance and *C. difficile* colitis.
- Follow isolation (respiratory or contact) precautions at all times, and wash your hands!

DRIPS

. . . And we're not talking about from your faucet . . .

- See ACLS section (Chapter 2) for IV drug doses.

TOTAL PARENTERAL NUTRITION (TPN)

. . . A viable GI tract is a terrible thing to waste . . .

- Consider this option if the GI tract is unusable for at least 7 days. Sterile vascular access is needed.
- Administered through the brown port of the triple lumen catheter. Reserve this port if you think initiating TPN is a possibility—cannot be used if it has been used previously.
- For initial orders and questions, a **nutritional support consult** will be valuable for information, advice, other options, and help with calculating projected nutritional needs.
- TPN orders must be written daily and received by a certain time—make sure this is done before signing out.
- Monitor vital signs, daily weight, I/Os, Accuchecks, and routine labs (CBC, electrolytes, BUN, SMA–9, Mg) frequently. Monitor triglycerides and hepatic function at least once a week.
- May add H_2 blockers, steroids, insulin, and vitamin K^+ to TPN if so desired.
- If TPN must be D/C'ed, monitor Accuchecks and administer IV fluids (e.g., D_{10}) at the same rate.

20

Final Touches

. . . Words to the wise and sleep deprived . . .

1. When in doubt, ask and ask again. Call someone (wake up someone if you need to), preferably someone who knows more than you do.
2. When in doubt, it's always better (albeit more painful) to go see the patient.
3. Listen to the patient.
4. The right thing to do usually involves less sleep.
5. Beware of those bearing scalpels.
6. Resist the temptation to discuss patient care in public areas; no good can come of it.
7. A healthy amount of compassion and compulsion makes it difficult to harm patients.
8. Help out your colleagues; they can return the favor when you need it most.
9. Walk if you don't need to run. Sit down if you don't need to walk. Lie down if there's a bed nearby. Answer all of nature's calls.
10. Residency, too, shall pass.

FEEDBACK

As this is the first edition of this guide, we are very interested in any comments you may have regarding making this guide more useful to its intended audience. Comments may be sent via electronic mail to wmisg@yahoo.com.

PATIENT DATA TRACKING FORM

Name:	
DOB	Age
Admitted	Discharged
Allergies	

HPI

PMH/PSH

Admission Meds

SH   FH

ROS

Admission

T	P	R	BP
O2		Wt	Ht

MCV=
RDW=

Ca		T bili		PTT			
Mg		D bili		PT			
Phos		AST		INR			
TP		ALT		Amylase			
Alb		Alk Ph		Lipase			

Previous Labs:

<u>EKG</u>   <u>CXR</u>

Admission: Admission:

Previous: Previous:

Previous Studies:

Problems:

Brief Course

Admission	Discharge
❑ Old data	❑ Placement
❑ Old records	
❑ DDx	❑ Home care
❑ Admit orders	
❑ Interview	❑ D/C orders
❑ H&P	
❑ Schedule tests	❑ Transport
❑ Read	
❑ DVT Proph	

Date								
Overnight Complaints								
	CP		SOB		CP		SOB	
	N/V		Abd		N/V		Abd	
	Urine		Ap/wt		Urine		Ap/wt	
	Fatig		BM		Fatig		BM	
	HA		Vis		HA		Vis	
	Aud				Aud			
Meds								
Relevant Tests								
T (Tmax)								
P								
R								
BP								
SaO$_2$								
I/O								
Accu								
Physical Exam								

Other Labs				
Tasks	❏ Pre-round ❏ Notes in chart ❏ Vitals ❏ Meds ❏ Labs ❏ Micro ❏ Note ❏ Order tests ❏ AM Labs	❏ Change meds ❏ Call consults ❏ Read consults ❏ Test results ❏ Chat with pt	❏ Pre-round ❏ Notes in chart ❏ Vitals ❏ Meds ❏ Labs ❏ Micro ❏ Note ❏ Order tests ❏ AM Labs	❏ Change meds ❏ Call consults ❏ Read consults ❏ Talk with other team members ❏ Test results ❏ Chat with pt and loved ones
A/P				

Index

Index

Notes